A MEDICAL TOUR THROUGH THE WHOLE
ISLAND OF GREAT BRITAIN

What kind of injuries do holidaymakers inflict on themselves on an awayday to Scarborough? Did the 'gene' for witchcraft come from a village in East Anglia? How can Ulster, despite decades of conflict, have a low rate of suicide? Did the spa at Bath really cure Royal infertility? Is Sellafield to blame for the leukaemia clusters in a neighbouring town?

Following in the footsteps of Daniel Defoe's *A Tour Through the Whole Island of Great Britain*, the psychiatrist Louis Appleby travels along the industrial, rural and coastal pathways of Great Britain and Northern Ireland. He discovers that illnesses do not arise spontaneously, but stem from the way people live and work, while medical treatments emerge not merely from science but from folklore, social fashion and political upheaval.

From the introduction of the Black Death to the spread of Aids, from Derbyshire Neck to the Dogger Bank Itch of Lowestoft fishermen, Louis Appleby reveals how the profile of Great Britain is written in its rich medical history.

Louis Appleby studied medicine in Edinburgh where he graduated in 1980. After postgraduate training in hospital medicine, he entered psychiatry in London and is now Senior Lecturer in Psychiatry at Manchester University. He has written for the *Observer*, *The Times* and the *New Statesman*, and contributes regularly to the Radio 4 mental health programme *All in the Mind*.

A Medical Tour
through the Whole Island of
Great Britain

LOUIS APPLEBY

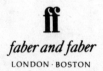

faber and faber
LONDON · BOSTON

First published in 1994
by Faber and Faber Limited
3 Queen Square London WC1N 3AU
This paperback edition first published in 1995

Photoset by Parker Typesetting Service, Leicester
Printed in England by Clays Ltd, St Ives plc

A CIP record for this book is available from the British Library

ISBN 0–571–17339–X

2 4 6 8 10 9 7 5 3 1

To JULIET and MICHELLE,
fellow travellers

Contents

INTRODUCTION

A Medical Tour

'It is not an easy thing to travel over a whole kingdom,' wrote Daniel Defoe in the second volume of *A Tour through the Whole Island of Great Britain*. For me, though, it was the only way of seeing what I had in mind – the facts and fables of British medicine and the places where they belonged. In viewing a country, as in caring at the bedside, the only sure way to know what is going on is to make the examination in person.

Medicine is a subject that sometimes seems to put up unnecessary barriers, to exclude outsiders and guard its own territory jealously. But the truth is that the boundaries that separate medicine and health from their cultural context are an invention: they do not really exist. Illnesses do not simply arise spontaneously: they are products of the way people live or where they work, and their treatments emerge not just from science but from folklore, social fashion and political upheaval.

As a result, the character of a country can be found in its pattern of illness and cure. The more varied the kingdom, the more diverse its diseases. And Britain, with its many types of race, trade and terrain, is a place where the medical mixture is rich.

I wanted to tour Great Britain and Northern Ireland with one broad question in mind: how does medicine fit into the larger map of the country, the cultural map made up of distinctive locations unique in their combination of history, religion, industry, myth and the lie of their land. I drew up plans to visit an inner city and an outer island, a seaside resort and a spa, a rural landscape and a fishing port, a coal-mine and a mill town. I set out to examine some of the major contemporary health controversies: Aids, the contamination of food, mental illness in immigrants, and the nuclear industry. This was to be a medical journey, a tour of health and ill health, and I hoped that local people and historical records would provide me with anecdotes and answers.

Anyone who tries to write about Britain is instantly aware of how many people have done it before and how well. But of the many authors who have travelled the country there were three to whom I found myself returning most often, three of the most English of writers, whose comments appear from time to time throughout this book. One is J. B. Priestley; the quotations are from his *English Journey*. Inevitably another is George Orwell, whose *Road to Wigan Pier* is referred to in the chapters on Wales and Bolton and whose *Down and Out in Paris and London* is the basis of the discussion with the Salvation Army in London.

The third is Daniel Defoe, whose *Tour* was a recurrent source of amusement and envy. Defoe had been to many of the places I visited, sometimes for the same reason. His book was a constant companion – and an encouragement, because Defoe was of the opinion that omissions and lost details in what was written were simply a reflection of the travel genre. According to him the private journey of the writer 'admits not the observer to dwell upon every nicety, to measure the distances, and determine exactly the site, the dimensions, or the extent of places, or read the histories of them'. There simply wasn't time to be so thorough. If this was his excuse for any mistakes, I was and still am happy to adopt it.

ONE

Dorset

NEAR where I was standing, between the ferry and the flooded quayside road, was the place where the plague entered Britain. At that time the ships mooring in Melcombe harbour came from across the English Channel and the west coast of France and it was one of these, said to be from Gascony, that delivered the infection. In fourteenth-century England diseases were bound to arrive that way. The island had its ports, the ports had ships, the ships had rats, the rats had fleas and the fleas carried the Black Death. Any trading nation could expect to import its epidemic.

I had reached Dorset the night before and slept in one of many hotels that took its name from the doomed hero of a Thomas Hardy novel; it occurred to me that Hardy wrote like a man who thought the plague would soon be back. In the morning I had driven to Weymouth which has long since swallowed Melcombe whole, though six centuries ago they were distinct towns on either side of the River Wey. The tourist office on the sea front was advertising a concert and a circus and the women ahead of me in the queue bought a pile of tickets. My turn came before I had worked out the best way to phrase my inquiry.

'What can you tell me about the Black Death?'

'What do you want to know?' The man at the desk gave me an impassive smile.

'Where exactly would it have come ashore?'

He wasn't sure, he told me. Probably near the mouth of the river on the Melcombe side, at the entrance to the old harbour. It seemed that no one knew the precise spot.

'So there's nothing there to celebrate it?'

'We're trying to forget it,' the tourist officer said with what looked like genuine shame.

Although it was not the first appearance of plague in England, the outbreak that began on the Dorset coast in June 1348 was the most catastrophic. By the end of the year it had spread throughout the South and within two years it had killed as many as 2 million people at a time when the entire country supported no more than 5 million and perhaps fewer. Villages were wiped out; the agricultural workforce was massacred. Nearly half the population died, the equivalent of 25 million deaths now.

I stood on the bridge that spans the Wey looking along the line of harbour buildings. On the day it happened there would have been a French sailing ship, probably an old inn and a crowd of men unloading the cargo that contained the lethal microbes. News of a terrible fever spreading across Europe would already have reached the seafaring towns along the south coast. But it would not have been called the Black Death, the name being a more recent invention, not heard in Britain at least until the seventeenth century; then, it seems to have been used to distinguish this epidemic from the Great Plague. To the people on the quay 600 years ago the ways of diseases were mysterious and the spread of the plague would have seemed an act of fate; where it would turn up was as unpredictable as the impact that it would soon have on the authority of both the Church and the landowning classes, both of which it undermined. And in a sense they were right: it was fate, or at least bad luck, that brought the infection here before any other port. Unseen and therefore unsuspected, the bacteria that shook the social order of the kingdom slipped into Melcombe. Fifty metres away, roughly where the schooner from Gascony would have moored, I could see a ship from Hamburg hoisting crates off its deck on to dry land; on the other side of the road there was a *health club*. This had to be the spot. Fate again.

Down Custom House Quay and along a narrow street I returned to the arc of sand that sweeps past the remnant of Melcombe Regis towards chalk cliffs further east. As the name showed, this was once a seaside patronized by royalty. George III took a plunge here and in doing so gave his imprimatur to the novel practice of sea bathing,

which was claimed to have medicinal value. Out of season this part of
the town seemed subdued and the hotels that stretched along the sea
front as far as I could see looked as if they were hibernating. It was a
place people retired to; men in fishermen's caps but with landlubbers'
faces were strolling beside the bay. The thin sunshine of late winter
and the clear sky made it the most invigorating of days.

I had come to Dorset to ask about animals and the diseases they
transmitted. Fears had been aroused around the country by reports of
infections carried to humans by animals on farms and in the wild.
There was controversy over salmonella in chickens; there were stories
of the spread of Weil's disease from rats and Lyme disease from deer;
most of all there had been alarm over bovine spongiform encephalopathy, which its alternative name of 'mad cow disease' had done
little to ease. A rural county like Dorset seemed the place to make
inquiries; with its acres of farm land it was where the food chain
started; its forests and streams sustained a rich wildlife. And, as I had
found out in Weymouth, it was still trying to live down its part in the
most horrifying condition caught from animals, bubonic plague. There
would be plenty to talk about when I met the district's expert on
infectious diseases.

I drove out of the town and for a couple of hours toured the narrow
lanes and villages around Dorchester, occasionally looking out for a
patch of ground overgrown enough to have been Hardy's model for
Egdon Heath, but every field seemed carefully kept. It is supposed that
the traditional English countryside owes much to the Black Death
because many of the ubiquitous hedgerows were built in its wake.
People died in such numbers between 1348 and 1350 that there were
often no surviving relatives to whom sick tenants could bequeath their
smallholdings. Land that became vacant in this way was sometimes
divided by landlords among those who owned neighbouring plots with
the result that the size of many holdings multiplied. Tenants who were
now in possession of substantial areas of cultivable ground chose to
mark out their territory, making their recent expansion clear to others,
and planted hedges along their borders.

The plague is also said to have led to a change in farming practice,
away from crops and towards sheep, the shortage of agricultural

workers caused by the epidemic making it easier to keep animals that could be left untended. But the evidence for a rapid rise in the sheep population is scarce. It seems more likely that the enormity of the Black Death led it to be credited with every social upheaval of the Middle Ages. Nevertheless, the area of Dorset where I was driving did gradually see a flourishing of livestock. When Daniel Defoe passed through in the early eighteenth century he was told that there were 600,000 sheep within six miles of Dorchester.

'Now and again we see a pregnant shepherdess who has to be advised not to help with the lambing,' Sarah Crook told me when we were seated in her office. 'It's in case she catches chlamydia from the sheep. But it means her job is on the line.' Despite the antiquated sound of 'pregnant shepherdesses' this is a modern danger to flocks and those who watch them. Chlamydia is the name given to a family of microscopic organisms that infect animals, one of its members producing psittacosis in parrots. A closely related species causes abortion among ewes by damaging the placenta; during the lambing season infection can spread to other sheep and pregnant women have been known to miscarry after catching it. The women's own health can also be seriously affected. 'I have personally seen two cases and one of them died,' said Dr Crook.

Sarah Crook's Dorchester workplace is an unmarked prefabricated building one storey high and, typical of public health departments, it is tucked at the edge of a residential street where no member of the public would look for it. Transmissible diseases in West Dorset are Dr Crook's speciality and I wanted to know about rats; now that the risk of plague in Britain had almost disappeared – though there was a limited outbreak in the early part of this century – did rats deserve their popular image as the most untouchable of vermin?

It is Weil's disease that the contemporary rat is accused of spreading, a potentially fatal jaundice resulting from infection with bacteria called leptospires, which are excreted in rat urine. Not everyone who catches the leptospire develops the same illness; in some people it provokes a fever, in others meningitis or kidney failure. Because of its connection with rats it is famous in medical circles as a disease of sewermen but, after the reputed rise in the number of rats inhabiting Britain's waterways, it is also said to present a risk to swimmers, canoeists and windsurfers.

But, said Sarah, the group of people most likely to pick up lepto-spirosis is none of these and the commonest animal source is no longer the rat. Of the fifty or so cases each year across the country, the majority come from cattle and occur in farmers. In the whole county of Dorset there are usually fewer than five cases each year; Dr Crook's most recent annual health records for West Dorset listed none at all. These are inauspicious days for the brown rat, a creature that seemed to me to be living on its reputation – or rather that of its predecessor in Britain, the black rat, which it replaced as the dominant species some time after the Great Plague. It is still feared, killed and shuddered at but its impact on health is small. Even as a cause of leptospirosis, its most characteristic contagion, it has been surpassed by the farmyard cow.

But there is one wild mammal known to harbour a human disease that is on the increase and unlike the rat it is an animal most people are pleased to encounter. In fact Lyme disease is not carried by deer themselves but by the ticks that feed off them, as the plague was by rat fleas. Usually those who acquire the responsible bug have only a mild illness but Lyme disease can progress, like syphilis (which is caused by a similar bacterium), from a simple rash and fever to an inflammation of the heart and nervous system. The first accounts of the condition were reported from Lyme, Connecticut, a town named by its original settlers after their ancestral home of Lyme Regis, a few miles from where we were in Dorchester; and it is rural, wooded counties such as Dorset that are likely to see most cases, the risk of infection in any area being proportionate to the number of deer that live there. In West Dorset the previous year had produced one con-firmed case, though Sarah thought there could have been many more that had come and gone unrecognized. In neighbouring Hampshire, twenty cases had occurred around the New Forest in the previous three years.

But, I wanted to know, how did the ticks attach themselves to people – presumably not straight from the deer. 'The ticks fall off and live in the grass,' explained Sarah, 'and then along come some walkers in shorts and they attach themselves to their legs and bite them. It isn't the local people who catch Lyme disease, it's the visitors; they are the ones who walk in tall grass with bare legs.'

It was a theme that she was quick to warm to: the way incomers to the rural scene fell ill while those who had always lived there did not. 'There's a misconception that people on the land suffer from exciting diseases they catch from animals.' I agreed: it was what I had thought. 'But a lot of them are immune.'

The same is true of cryptosporidium, a life-form about the size of an amoeba, to which it is distantly related. The illness that results from swallowing it is a kind of gastro-enteritis; the diarrhoea is sometimes severe enough to necessitate fluid replacement by intravenous tube. In calves and lambs it produces a similar condition known as scours and these animals have been blamed for infecting humans and causing a peak in incidence around lambing time. There has also been one recorded outbreak among schoolchildren on an educational visit to an Oxfordshire farm. Yet farm workers themselves rarely suffer from it and appear to build up an immunity through repeated exposure to the organism.

The other way to catch cryptosporidium is to drink it in unpasteurized milk or contaminated water. 'I feel strongly about untreated milk,' said Sarah. 'It isn't just cryptosporidium. It can contain salmonella and campylobacter. But in a dairy county like Dorset it is drunk a lot. You can't sell it but it can be given free to tourists who are staying in a farmhouse bed and breakfast. The local people drink it but they don't get ill because they've developed a resistance. Yet if you try to restrict it and make people use pasteurized milk, they protest. It's not just a medical issue; if it affects the business of renting cottages to holiday-makers, it's about their livelihood. And it limits their freedom. Untreated milk is politically sensitive stuff. And unfortunately people say it tastes better.'

Salmonella has long been the main culprit in the thousands of cases of gastro-enteritis in Britain every year but in 1990 campylobacter overtook it. Until the 1970s it was little more than a bacteriological curiosity because under the microscope it has an odd spiral appearance. It was not at that time considered to be a significant source of illness in humans although it was known to exist in the intestines of many animals, including livestock. Now it is held responsible for over 30,000 cases of diarrhoea every year, some of these in outbreaks of hundreds. Any reservoir is at risk of receiving it through animal urine but Dr Crook sees private water supplies as a greater problem.

'Private supplies can be full of bacteria but the people who have used them for years are not harmed by them. Then they rent out their houses to visitors with babies and there's an outbreak of infection. Private water is like untreated milk. It's common in Dorset. Only in the case of water there are new regulations and people will have to change. They object because they've never been ill themselves and they're worried about the expense of a new water system. They're immune. They don't see living close to animals as a threat to their health.'

Benjamin Jesty would have been intrigued to hear this talk of immunity, but not surprised. Earlier in the day I had driven to his birthplace, Yetminster, and then to his grave in Worth Matravers. It seemed a rather hasty way of looking over a man's existence. But Jesty's eulogists would say that his life had always been unjustly ignored, because it was he, they insist, and not the celebrated Edward Jenner, who discovered vaccination.

Yetminster is an old village that has sprouted new side-streets where clusters of modern houses stretch the original boundary. I turned off what appeared to be the main village road and drove up the hill to where St Andrew's Church stood beside buildings labelled in a way that emphasized their age. There was the Old Vicarage, the Old Rectory and the Old School. Yetminster was keen to make it clear how much it valued tradition over progress. Benjamin Jesty would not have been surprised by this either.

Not far from the Old Church was the site of Upbury Farm, where Jesty was living when he carried out the first known vaccination in Britain; in 1774 he injected his wife and sons with fluid infected with cowpox in the hope of saving them from smallpox. This was not as reckless as it sounds: smallpox was sweeping Dorset with its usual combination of high mortality and public terror and desperate measures would have seemed worth the risk.

As bubonic plague had declined in the late seventeenth century, smallpox had taken its place, arriving in regular epidemics that killed thousands. It was not a new disease, having become common in the sixteenth century when it had struck Elizabeth I, leaving her pock-marked and bald but nevertheless alive. But it does seem to have become more aggressive: Queen Mary, the wife of William III, died of it during an epidemic in 1694 – William himself was also infected – and throughout the next hundred years its incidence grew until it was widespread and lethal enough to be one of the main restrictions on the growth of the country's population.

The mark of the disease was small blisters of fluid, rich in the smallpox virus, which peppered the skin of feverish victims. A similar blister also occurred on the udders of cattle with cowpox, a much milder condition that impaired the quality of milk. Cowpox could be passed on to humans if the fluid from these pustules came into contact with broken skin during milking, so many farmers and their employees caught the disease and developed blistered hands and sometimes a raised temperature. In Dorset and neighbouring counties there was a tradition that anyone who had picked up cowpox could not also go down with smallpox and it is supposedly for this reason that milkmaids, whose immunity prevented their faces from becoming pock-marked, were habitually described as 'fair' in songs and rural mythology.

Jesty was a farmer in his thirties when the 1774 outbreak of smallpox reached Yetminster. Several deaths followed in the village but on his farm the cowpox legend must have seemed plausible. Not only did Jesty himself remain unaffected but so did two farm hands, Ann Notley and Mary Reade, who in addition to their duties at Upbury, were now nursing relatives with smallpox who lived nearby. All three had had cowpox and Jesty must have been confident of its protective power to allow the two women to divide their time between victims of the disease and his young family. And when he heard that cowpox had broken out at a farm two miles away at Chetnole he decided to provide his wife and two sons, though for some reason not his infant daughter, with the same protection.

At the contaminated farm Jesty collected pus from one of the available udders, made a scratch on his wife's arm with a darning needle and rubbed in the cowpox. He did the same with the two boys.

they are more likely to be found in cases of food poisoning. In the ten years from 1980 the number of cases of salmonella occurring annually in England and Wales tripled to over 30,000. Two recent outbreaks in West Dorset were typical of how the illness can be spread. The first had affected three people at a private buffet; the food there had been prepared by someone who was found to be a carrier, loaded with salmonella but free of symptoms. The other was believed to have been caused by contaminated eggs.

Most microbiologists would agree that poultry and eggs are the most frequent source of food poisoning in the UK, although meat and raw milk are responsible for some cases, and that *Salmonella* species are often to blame. Studies in the 1980s found these bacteria in about two-thirds of fresh and frozen chickens. I asked Sarah what she thought.

'I think,' she said deliberately, 'that there's a problem.'

'With the chicken or the egg?'

'The type of *Salmonella* is the same so you can't tell what proportion of cases is caused by each of them individually. Everyone has been suspicious about eggs for years but the problem with eggs will be there until salmonella is eliminated from the farm breeding stock. While the grandfather chickens still have it, the number of cases can carry on increasing.'

So that was clear enough: the fears were reasonable. But if popular unease over salmonella was high, it was nothing compared to the anxiety engendered by bovine spongiform encephalopathy. Dismissed as hysteria by some, justified by critics of modern food production, the reaction to a disease which had never been found in humans was as extraordinary as the condition itself.

In fact BSE had never been reported at all until 1987 but within three years almost twenty thousand cases had been confirmed in Britain. Infected cattle developed odd movements and their mental faculties degenerated. It was universally fatal and at post-mortem holes were found in their brains, hence the name. It appeared to result from infection by an organism similar to a virus but hardier, as it was able to withstand any sterilization technique from boiling to irradiation.

But what really caused panic was that the disease was similar to a condition of sheep known as scrapie, so called because affected animals scrape themselves against fence posts to relieve itching. This raised the possibility that BSE had been transmitted to cows by feeding them on meat and bone meal from sheep that had been carrying scrapie; and in support of this theory it was then discovered that by this route mink on farms in the USA had acquired an identical neurological illness. If the infection could pass between animal species, could it also affect humans? There were two reasons to think it might: Creutzfeld-Jakob disease and kuru. The first is a rare disorder causing twitching movements and dementia which can be infective, though the micro-organism has never been found. Kuru is a medical oddity, a fatal disease of the nervous system once found in a cannibalistic tribe in Papua New Guinea whose men ate the muscle of corpses while the women consumed the remaining scraps including the brain. Almost all cases of kuru were women. Perhaps these diseases – which may actually be the same thing – were the human equivalent of BSE and perhaps the mad cow virus could infect humans. If so, those who ate meat products made from beef offal could be imperilled. But if there was a threat from beef, why had the disease not already been passed on to people who ate its original host species, the sheep? I asked Sarah if she thought human infection was possible.

'You can't say,' she hedged. 'There isn't enough evidence to decide. There has never been a case; but on the other hand several other species have been infected in laboratory tests, including monkeys.'

'Do people on farms worry about it?'

'They worry because it affects their business. Diseases like BSE alter customers' eating habits. There's less demand for beef.' As with the milk, there were no fears for illness, just fears for income. Mad cow disease is a hypothetical medical threat but a real economic hazard; yet it has been able to get under the skin of our culture and revive the most acute terror of disease. Everything about it is disturbing. It causes madness. Its effect is delayed; years may go by before it makes its sinister presence evident. It may already be in the food chain, waiting to turn our brains *spongiform*, a nightmarish word conjuring up an image of brain tissue full of holes through which our sanity drains away. It is no wonder that a condition that has yet to claim a single victim has picked up such a malevolent reputation.

But there is another reason for all the disquiet over BSE and that is its animal origin: it seemed to me that it was following a tradition begun by the diseases I had heard about earlier that day. Some of our most horrific illnesses – bubonic plague and rabies are examples – have been caught from animals which have come to represent an especially dangerous source of sickness. BSE has stirred up an ancient ingrained fear. There is also an impression that the feeding practices that seem to have encouraged it to jump from one creature to another, the practices that allow sheep to be fed to cows, are unnatural. This threat from more primitive creatures comes from a disturbance of the established order and, as Benjamin Jesty learned, that is something our species does not easily tolerate.

By the time I left Sarah Crook's office it was late afternoon but I had planned a short detour before heading out of Dorset. At Maiden Newton, a few miles to the north, I turned off the main road and drove along a thin lane until I came across a farm, a row of cottages and a bulky house in its own grounds. This was Wynford Eagle, where Thomas Sydenham was born in 1624.

Sydenham became one of the country's most influential doctors but when he lived here he was a soldier, a junior member of a family of cantankerous men who supported Cromwell and who were known in the locality as 'the fighting Sydenhams'. There were two reasons for their opposition to the Royalists: first, they were Puritans; second, they resented the amount that they and the rest of Dorset had to pay the king in taxes. When the Civil War came they joined the Dorset militia and Thomas's brother William became a colonel and a close battle-field companion to Sir Anthony Ashley Cooper, the first Earl of Shaftesbury.

Of the six Sydenham brothers who fought against the king's men, two – Francis and John – were killed. William survived and was made Governor of Weymouth. Thomas, who served as a cornet, an officer rank with the high-profile responsibility of carrying the colour, was wounded three times. On one occasion, probably at the Battle of

Worcester, he was left for dead. In 1646 he had seen enough of war and took up medicine, a decision that would lead him into a more sedate rebellion, against the medical theories that had prevailed for centuries.

I stopped my car and peered into the grounds of the large house. Was this the descendant of the manor house where the Sydenhams had lived? A woman came out, eyed me suspiciously and shot back inside. I decided not to ask her; this did not seem the right moment. In any case, Thomas Sydenham's triumphs as a doctor happened not here but in central London. I could pick up his trail later.

TWO

Bristol and Bath

THE ROAD through Clifton vanished into the drizzle, swerved and climbed past shop fronts and jutting side-streets, past wooded gardens and polite hotels and tall, opulent terraces, rose and opened briefly on to parkland that tilted back towards the town, before leaving the contour to its abrupt fall, a sudden plunge of a hundred metres to where the Avon, swollen by the rain, eroded the mud along the belly of the gorge. Above the river, piercing the downpour, stood the Clifton Suspension Bridge, an engineering colossus spanning the ravine where it has witnessed more than a century of suicides, a monument to ingenuity and a symbol of desperation.

People who seem to be thinking of suicide can sometimes be seen taking a look at the bridge, eyeing the drop, checking out their method and their nerve. I parked and walked up the grass slope. Afterwards I thought I remembered a sign warning drivers that there was no turning back once they had reached the slip road to the toll-booth. But it may simply have been an impression left by the bridge itself. From here there was no going back.

From a roadside bench a man in his thirties glanced at me, then went back to studying the ground between his knees. He looked like someone waiting for his own gallows to open but whatever he was thinking, he was startled out of it by a sudden shriek from the bridge, then several more. It was a false alarm, just a crowd of back-packed, back-slapping Spanish teenagers who were shouting and shoving each other around the walkway.

At the toll-booth pedestrians paid two pence to walk across: I had the macabre thought of would-be suicides forgetting to bring some change. It was not as unlikely as it sounded. Small obstacles have been known to prevent that most enormous of acts, self-annihilation. There is one suicide bridge where barbed wire trailed along the top of a barrier led fewer people to clamber over, as if all that was needed to make oblivion less attractive was that extra inconvenience.

There is also the case of the young woman who leaped off the Clifton Suspension Bridge a hundred years ago but whose petticoats were inflated by the wind, causing her to parachute daintily to the ground. You might think her response would have been the most intense frustration, that she might have ripped off her undergarments, stalked out of the gorge and grimly jumped again. She didn't. She went home, never tried to repeat her attempt and lived into her eighties.

Enough is known about what makes people kill themselves to fill a library. Suicide rates are higher in men and increase with age. Divorce, unemployment, and bereavement add to the risk. So do alcoholism and mental illness in all its varieties. Everything is clear on the subject except the final motivation. What is the difference between the moment before a suicidal thought and the moment it arises? Between the day of watching the bridge and the day of jumping? There are those who think about suicide every morning for thirty years, then one day they do it. Why then?

Anyone who claims to know the whole answer to this question is bound to be wrong but one component of the suicidal impulse is known. Part of this uniquely human act is the uniquely human capacity to expect the future: the same awareness of tomorrow that makes someone invest his money or plan a holiday also lies behind his act of self-destruction, because the mental characteristic on which suicide finally relies is loss of hope.

Like murder, suicide needs both motive and opportunity and wherever river bridges have been erected, from Brisbane to the Golden Gate, people have seen their chance and jumped. But not just any people. Jumping to certain death is a young person's act and an insane person's act. It is rarely a lover's leap; it is seldom so romantic. Violent suicides, on bridges as on railway tracks, are isolated men of thirty or forty. Or they are psychotic, egged on by relentless voices from the air.

Although the pocket guidebook on sale at the toll kiosk did not mention the Clifton Suspension Bridge's reputation for suicide, it is one that was quickly earned. Isambard Kingdom Brunel's design was itself the result of a brush with death in which his father's tunnel under the Thames caved in on him during 1828. Convalescing in the West Country, Brunel was drawn to the engineering challenge of the Avon gorge but lack of money delayed the construction until 1864, five years after his death. Two years later, the first person jumped.

Even though people have been leaping from the bridge ever since, the suicide rate in Bristol is no higher than in any other British town. This may simply reflect the relative rarity of the river bridge method; it would take a huge spate of bridge suicides to inflate the overall total. It could also be that methods of suicide, rather than rates, are the best reflection of the geography and character of a society; there are many illustrations of the way national habits can influence suicidal actions. In the USA, for example, young men often kill themselves violently, just as they do here, but mainly with that American symbol, the gun. Similarly, when natural gas replaced the more toxic town gas in the UK's domestic supply in the 1960s, the country's suicide rate declined; the gas oven method had become less dependable.

Of all the routes to self-destruction, the commonest in contemporary Britain did not exist when the Clifton Bridge was built. Drugs prescribed by doctors are taken by many of the five thousand who kill themselves annually and though complex motives lead people to destroy themselves with something given to help them, this fact too is an illustration of the way in which suicide is a mirror held up to the surrounding culture. Medicine has claimed, or at least accepted, distress as its own domain and many people trying to stop themselves from ending their lives would turn to a doctor for help. The fact that doctors are also the people who provide the method can be seen as a reflection, admittedly a distorted one, of their role as comforters.

If despair and a convenient method were all that suicide required, it would be a puzzle that so few people go through with it. Five thousand each year is only 1 per cent of deaths in Britain and it is not perverse to ask what stops all the others who ever consider it from going ahead. Put that question to individuals who are depressed and the replies are surprisingly consistent. Religion is a common reason, as is concern for children. Some say it is fear of pain that holds them back. Some say it is fear of not succeeding.

But there may be another reason, a paradoxical reason, in what I learned in Clifton. If despair grows out of the feeling that events are out of control and if suicide is an escape from despair, then suicide in a few cases at least is a method of reasserting the control that has been lost. It therefore seems possible that viewing the bridge, by confirming that the method of suicide is there for when it is needed, could help a desperate person to feel back in control of his future and thereby lessen the urge to use it.

I wandered across the ravine in both directions until I was wetter than I wanted to be, then waded towards my car. The bench beside the road was now empty and I wondered for a moment what the solitary man had been thinking and what decision he had made.

Downhill from the bridge and half a century before it was built, a cardsharp and chemist-turned-doctor, Thomas Beddoes, set up his clinic for the experimental use of inhalation to treat consumption. As a student in Edinburgh in the 1780s, Beddoes found himself caught up in the swirl of scientific interest in newly discovered gases such as oxygen and hydrogen. Although he was there to train in medicine, he preferred chemistry classes and is credited with demonstrating the lifting strength of 'hydrogen in a glazed envelope', meaning the hydrogen balloon.

If it had not been for his inability to keep quiet on the hot politics of the day, Beddoes might have been lost to medicine, remaining instead a reader in pneumatic chemistry in Oxford, the post he occupied on completing his medical studies. As it was, he spoke out against the Indian empire, for the French Revolution and the rights of man, and quite clearly against William Pitt, a liberal stance that forced his resignation. So in 1793, while Pitt was entering a war with France, Beddoes was opening his Pneumatic Institute in Dowry Square, Clifton, and pioneering the 'medicinal use of factitious airs'.

By applying modern science to medical practice he hoped to cure one of the deadliest of diseases, tuberculosis. Pulmonary consumption, its most lethal form, was common in cities such as Bristol. Its victims coughed and sweated, their lungs devoured by abscesses, scars and cavities, one of which might finally burst in the bloody climax that became almost a tradition for the romantic heroine. There was no treatment that worked and it would be several decades before the bacteria that cause TB were shown even to exist.

Beddoes believed the new gases carried a therapeutic potential which went beyond consumption to scrofula – a tuberculous infection of lymph glands in the neck – and on to such disparate conditions as opium addiction and catarrh. He designed what was in effect a proto-type of the oxygen tent and experimented with anything from oxygen to carbon monoxide.

In his laboratory work he was assisted by a young Humphry Davy for whom this was the start of a lifelong fascination with the properties of gases. Davy was one of those scientists whose interest in his subject was so intense that he recklessly used himself as a test subject, on one occasion almost asphyxiating in an attempt to understand the effects of nitrous oxide. After that he stuck to recording the reactions of other people, of whom there was no shortage as the fame of the Pneumatic Institute travelled. Regular volunteers included Robert Southey and Samuel Taylor Coleridge, who were part of a poetic coterie living it up in Bristol at the time.

Coleridge, his career as an opium addict still ahead of him, was an admirer of this putative cure and its inventor. His account of how it felt to breathe nitrous oxide was jotted down by Davy beside the descrip-tions of less illustrious guinea-pigs and led ultimately to the most enduring discovery of the Beddoes–Davy partnership: the rapid ni-trous oxide anaesthesia which they publicized in 1799 and which is still in widespread use.

Southey too enjoyed inhalation and often went back for more. He once wrote to his brother Tom that nitrous oxide 'made me laugh and tingle in every toe and finger-tip'. He even praised the black bladder through which the vapour was delivered, calling it 'oh excellent air-bag'. In the end the exponents of the new treatment overdid the eulogies. Although Beddoes was determined that the discovery would be put to medicinal use, nitrous oxide was soon better known as laughing gas and did not enter surgical practice in Britain until 1868, by which time both ether and chloroform had been in use for more than twenty years.

In 1803 Beddoes transferred his activities to the centre of Bristol, off Broad Quay, under a new name, the Preventive Medicine Institution. By now he was combating infection on more than one front, examining the healthy families of consumptives for signs of incipient disease, and identifying high-risk trades, such as stone-cutting. His advice included good diet, rest and warmth; he once told a sick farmer to move into his barn, where the heat of his animals would be beneficial.

But his far-sightedness ruffled medical orthodoxy and in the eyes of his peers Beddoes now crossed the line that separates innovator from eccentric. Nor were the citizens of Bristol slow to brand his methods as disreputable or to spread a story that one of the gases he recommended was the breath of a cow. Popular opinion became so uniformly hostile that his *modus operandi* came to signify the depths of quackery which some doctors were ready to plumb. In 1805 a public debate, on whether doctors should be allowed to attend operations on people other than their own patients, led a city newspaper to publish a letter about the dangers of an unrestricted profession. 'What security have you,' asked the letter, 'that your wards shall not be turned into cow houses and your apothecary shop into a manufactory of gases?'

Three years later, at the age of forty-eight, Beddoes was dead. When Coleridge heard the news, he wept uncontrollably and later claimed that 'more hope has been taken out of my life by this than by any former event'. He had succumbed to a suppurating contagion which had attacked his lungs and heart. It was not tuberculosis and the traditional 'boiling blister' treatment, intended to draw out internal infection, proved useless, as Beddoes himself might have expected.

From Broad Quay I walked north past monuments and streets that jogged the memory of Bristol's heyday. Famous sons, native and (more often) adopted, were all there on a plaque or a pedestal, from the Cabots to Edmund Burke to Neptune. It seemed great men had only to ask the way out of town to reappear as a statue.

Bristol boasts too of embodying that most withering of urban insults, 'provincial', a word which the town's history has imbued with something admirable: autonomy and distinctness of identity. To tourists such as J. B. Priestley, Bristol was a model provincial capital, proud of its native entrepreneurs; they had exploited its position facing west, or more precisely the West Indies, and created a lucrative trade triangle to take cargo, some of it human, between England, West Africa and the Caribbean.

Tobacco, alcohol and chocolate, the demons of modern health care, made Bristol rich but the abolition of slavery sent the city into decline. Over a century later, when the descendants of West African slaves travelled the second side of the triangle, they set up home where decline was most in evidence, the inner city, a phrase that ends naturally with 'deprivation' or, as in the case of St Paul's in Bristol, 'riots'.

'We have to keep saying inner cities so that people will listen,' Stefan Cembrowicz told me. His inner-city general practice, covering St Paul's and the adjacent district of Montpelier, receives a deprivation allowance on as many as one-fifth of its patients because of the extra health care which poverty demands. Inner cities themselves may be crumbling but the term is fashionable and spawns easy platitudes, as does 'multicultural'. About 30 per cent of Dr Cembrowicz's patients are first- or second-generation immigrants and most of these come from the West Indies. The others are refugees of successive foreign crises: from Vietnam, Uganda, Hungary and 1940s Poland, from where Stefan's father escaped as a student after his room-mate was shot by the NKVD, the forerunners of the KGB.

I found St Paul's in gregarious mood: today was carnival. At the mouth of each road into its centre shuffled a group of policemen with the pallid, sunken look that goes with community-consciousness. Among them there was a bloated man in a straw hat which seemed to have been used to make his moustache. The word SECURITY on his lapel could be read a street away.

Most of the partying locals, decked out in Jamaican colours, pretended to ignore the police; the rest weren't pretending. On garden walls they sprawled, as if left there by the swell of the crowd. From huge speakers at the corner of Grosvenor Road, a deafening off-beat blasted the populace, submerging the fizz of beer cans and the distant competition of religious steel bands.

When Stefan Cembrowicz tried to drive through the same street one day in 1980, three burning police cars, one on top of the other, blocked his way. Nevertheless the first St Paul's riot, visible beyond the barricades, looked surprisingly good-humoured, almost like a carnival. But when the riots recurred six years later, the atmosphere was bitter. In a drugs raid no fewer than 600 police had been employed to cordon off part of the district – an unnecessary show of force, Stefan believed. Outraged young blacks were soon on the streets smashing windows and setting fires. In the middle of this mayhem, shortly before 3 a.m., Dr Cembrowicz received an emergency call from an estate in the middle of the trouble.

'An elderly Chinese man was unable to pass urine,' he told me. 'I remember thinking that this was urgent. I would have to get there despite the difficulties.' There were Landrovers across the entrance to St Paul's, put in place by the police who were unsure what to expect. 'I could hear glass breaking a street or two away. I asked the police if it was safe to go in but no one seemed to know.'

Grosvenor Road was in thick darkness; there was no street lighting, no light in any window and no number on any door. Stefan edged his way round gardens, peering and trying to guess where his patient lived. 'Suddenly six black teenagers appeared from nowhere. They were very excited and jumpy. We stood there looking at each other and one of them said, "Let's scalp him".'

Stefan slowed down his practised narrative to step up the irony: 'I tried to tell myself I was still at an advantage. If I used my superior education, I could get out of this fix. But somehow . . . nothing came to mind. Then another of the teenagers yelled, "It's Dr Stefan! It's OK, he's cool!" I think I had treated his mother at one time. They were obviously relieved. They said, "You should be more careful, Doc. It's not safe here. There's a lot of police around."'

The gang joined Stefan in his search. When they found the house, it too was in darkness and had to be woken up, though the elderly Chinaman was not easy to rouse. Having waited as long as he could, he had smoked a heap of opium and fallen into a painless sleep.

White visitors to St Paul's Festival came in every variety of the species. Evangelists, spare-time sociologists, families with push-chairs and whistles mingled around the stalls and stages. And away from them, mistrustfully apart, squatting in ragged circles, young whites in combat jackets and facsimile-dreadlocks, the whites in black disguise, copying their brothers in disillusionment.

Nowhere in the rows of kiosks and self-help societies that I browsed past was there any mention of the health controversy which centres on the black ghettos and embodies every element of urban and racial disadvantage. You could find out what you wanted to know about sickle cell disease, you could join Black Women for Wages for Housework, you could complain at the local authority information desk – its placard read 'Trouble with landlords? Problems with rats?' But you could only stay in the dark about schizophrenia.

For sixty years, studies of immigrants have turned up high rates of serious mental illness. The first was the work of a Norwegian alienist (as psychiatrists were then known) called Odegaard who watched with an opportunist's eye as his countrymen migrated to the American Midwest, where they settled from Minneapolis to Lake Wobegon. Dr Odegaard discovered more mental illness in migrant Norwegians than in those who stayed put and he wrote a pioneering treatise entitled 'Emigration and insanity' to demonstrate the point. But what did his findings prove?

One explanation was that the stress of migration provoked insanity, the other was that insane people, or at least those most likely to become insane, were also most likely to migrate. A third possibility, one that attracted less support in arguments between the other two, was that both might be correct.

The debate survived an inert period in the history of psychiatry when the presumed causes of mental illness were challenged, as was the concept itself. Schizophrenia, it was argued, was a way of relating to the world as valid as the 'sane' way and perhaps more insightful. Or it was a product of disjointed families or cock-eyed parenting. Or it was caused by the institutions that claimed to treat it. These theories could have left mental health for years in a scientific backwater.

Instead they forced on psychiatric research an experimental rigour which, in proving them to be nonsense, boosted understanding of mental illness in ways which are central to the dispute surrounding immigration.

No one who knows anything about it now doubts that schizophrenia is a brain disease and the only serious alternative to this view is that it is several brain diseases of similar appearance. Its commonest features are delusional ideas, often of being under threat, and hallucinations, usually in the form of imagined voices, but it also leads to a loss of higher mental abilities such as motivation, emotional responsiveness and richness of thought. It is, at least some of the time, inherited as a vulnerability to episodes of illness which are then triggered by environmental stress. In some cases the vulnerability may be minor brain damage arising at or before birth. So, if immigrants do suffer more from schizophrenia, are they more vulnerable and are they more stressed?

A common tactic in medicine, when it is struggling to come up with an answer, is to reassess the question. The immigration question is flawed because it is several questions masquerading as one. Immigrants are not a uniform collection of people, their reasons for migrating are various, their fortunes in their new countries differ. Even in a single country like Britain, there is no single experience of immigration. The Poles who reached Britain in the 1940s, Stefan Cembrowicz's father among them, were escapees from their homeland, relieved to be here and received as allies. Already educated, they made a success of their adopted home and merged with its inhabitants. The West Indians who arrived in St Paul's thirty years ago were different on every count.

In the UK, questions of immigration are about race or, more precisely, colour, and mental health questions are no exception. High rates of mental illness have been found in most immigrant groups, particularly West Africans and West Indians, and the same explanations considered by Odegaard are still put forward. Perhaps early mental illness makes people restless or fearful until they set off for another country. Or else those who are socially disadvantaged, some of them mentally vulnerable, seek work in whatever country offers it, as Britain did in the early 1960s. Or it could be that the stress of setting up a new life in an alien culture is just too great for some.

Any of these, or any combination of them, could be the reason for the excess of schizophrenia in first-generation immigrants. But what they do not explain is something even more alarming, something Odegaard would not have predicted: the even higher rates of schizophrenia reported in second-generation West Indian immigrants living in some of Britain's cities, rates which reach scarcely believable levels, over ten times the rate in the indigenous whites.

If questions of immigration are about race, then equally, questions of race are soon about racism. Academic arguments over the findings – and there have been plenty – have been overshadowed by racial sensitivity, which all sides claim, and accusations of racism, universally denied. To say that a racial minority is prone to mental illness, so claims the most extreme criticism, is a medical way of saying it is mentally weak. After all, the distinction of lunacy from mental enfeeblement is a new fashion, made clear only during this century.

Even more bitter is the comparison with the fracas twenty years ago over race and intelligence in which psychology became enmeshed under the hypocritical cloak of scientific objectivity; it reported results suggesting that blacks had lower IQs on average than whites. Unpalatable truths are no less true because they are unpalatable, it was imperiously claimed by some academics who should, and probably did, know better. But their findings were quickly attacked on the grounds that it was economics and education that determined scores on IQ tests rather than race; the tests of intelligence carried a cultural bias; and IQ itself was an invented concept: a way of looking at people, not an innate quality. The only conclusion to be drawn, then? Never, but never, trust an experimenter who confuses test results with truth.

But racism among researchers is not likely in the debate about schizophrenia: the dispute is not about an artificial concoction like IQ but something unmistakeable, madness. True, severe mental illness is perceived in different ways according to ethnic setting but everywhere it is found – which is everywhere anyone has looked – it is bad news. So, unlike IQ but like wisdom, it is not a creation of one culture imposed on another. All societies suffer it, recognize it and treat it, although in some countries the treatment may be no more than a rope with a tree at the other end.

A more likely mistake in studying other races is cultural ignorance and its consequence, racial stereotyping. The anthropological overview – the name anthropologists give to their own opinions – asserts that, while disturbed behaviour may exist in every culture, to call some of it illness is to apply a western idea where it is not useful. By this line of thought, the danger in districts such as St Paul's is mistaken labelling so that all reactions to stress are seen as mental disorder and all mental disorders are seen as schizophrenia.

If this attack sounds familiar, it is because it echoes the earlier objections to the concept of mental illness, the same attack that nearly damaged psychiatry beyond repair. The themes are the same: it isn't illness, just behaviour; it doesn't need treatment, just understanding. In any case the so-called treatment is a deception, runs the anti-psychiatry argument; it is social control wearing a white coat, the established order oppressing a minority of which it knows and sees nothing.

But none of this fits the facts. It is not in an isolated immigrant group, cocooned in its own world, that the highest rates of schizophrenia have been found. It is in young Afro-Caribbeans, who are partly integrated into white culture. And this no man's land which they inhabit may be the point, composed as it is of ramshackle estates and barren job centres.

As with Minnesota's Norwegians, so with Britain's blacks: are the pressures of being an immigrant to blame, or were the migrants prone to breakdown, or both? If there is a racial error in the debate, it lies in not accepting the *possibility* that some races in Britain are more susceptible than others, even though the question why is unanswered. According to the economic incentive theory, the early 1960s could have invited a genetically vulnerable migrant, one who was struggling to keep a job in Jamaica but who was promised one here. Then there is the infection theory: maybe the babies of migrants were uniquely sensitive to a virus with the power to damage embryonic brains slightly but crucially, with the effect that the second generation is more prone to the illness. Both theories are plausible, both unprovable.

But if the nature of any vulnerability is obscure, the stresses which act upon it are not hard to find in St Paul's: bad housing, no jobs, a generation trapped in a limbo between two cultures. And then there is racism. Racism, no one can doubt, contributes to the inflated figures for mental breakdown in young blacks but not because doctors are racist or because medical thinking is riddled with it. It is at the root of the economic misery, humiliating white abuse and heavy-handed policing of the kind that preceded the riots in Bristol in the mid-1980s.

The rates of schizophrenia in young blacks may not turn out to be quite as high as people now fear. Stefan Cembrowicz doubts it, from the numbers in his own practice. But they are certainly too high for the luxury of prolonged rumination, which is why Bristol has created its own mental health unit ostensibly for the inner city, based in Montpelier. What it really does is provide for the health of the run-down black estates, although to say so openly is considered bad form, a reminder of the stigma which mental illness still attracts.

St Paul's was running into serious rain by the time I had walked the length of its carnival and loitered round its low-lying flats. The crowds were still growing, shuffling and dancing, and Red Stripe tins still flashed. A man of twenty in a mac that didn't fit was holding out a leaflet called 'How to become a Christian' and thriving on refusal. From the back of the nearest lorry songs were being dedicated to God and Malcolm X in turn.

The festival had presented, side by side, the origins of the ill health I had wanted to explore and a hint of its remedy. The district looked poor as parts of all towns look poor but it looked something else, which the fluorescence of the street party emphasized. It looked colourless, which is another way of saying it looked hopeless and, as the Clifton Bridge had reminded me, nothing is more damaging to a society or the individuals within it than loss of hope.

Race in the inner cities is as much a health issue as it is one of economics or xenophobia. Culture-sensitive health care is one answer, dispassionate study of the facts is another, but the epidemic of psychosis in Afro-Caribbeans needs a solution to the failure of cultural assimilation which forces blacks into white society where they wind up at its lower end. This is a mental health crisis with a social remedy: a genuinely hybrid culture that goes beyond the superficiality of the white man's dreadlocks.

Threading my way out of the city centre, I was aware that serious arguments can, as time passes, sound like empty slogans.

The steady rain left me only a hazy view of Brislington House, a warehouse-breadth away from the last of Bristol's industrial suburbs on the Bath road. If the journey through Avon had something optimistic to reveal about mental illness, this was it, the site of a triumph for Thomas Beddoes's contemporary, Edward Long Fox.

Like those other reformers of the lunatic asylum, the Tuke family of York, Fox was a Quaker and it was thanks to his religious pacifism that he first discovered the thrill of notoriety. On completing his medical training in 1781 he joined his father Joseph in practice in Falmouth and walked straight into a public dispute over the latest skirmishes with France. Joseph Fox ran a sideline in merchant shipping and in the maritime free-for-all that the fighting allowed he could have pocketed £22,000, his share of the loot that his ships plundered from French vessels. But on principle he gave it all back to its rightful owners, except for £120 which went unclaimed.

Edward volunteered to be the agent of reparation and even travelled to France to hand over the money in person. Falmouth's local newspaper remarked that, apart from the nation's enemies, only his patients would applaud his trip: while he was away they could expect to enjoy good health. Undeterred, he went on to set up a charity for wounded French seamen using the final £120.

Within a few years he was working as a physician in Bristol where he pronounced scathingly on the popular treatments of the day. These included potions straight from the blasted heath, such as crab's eyes and pulverized toad, but also such elaborate remedies as hot, split pigeon – applied as a poultice to the soles of the feet. Fox theorized on what he called the 'animalcular origin' of diseases and in doing so may have anticipated the discoveries of Pasteur, Lister and John Snow, whose genius in the matter of a Soho water pump I was planning to explore when I reached central London.

At the same time he championed the cause of prisoners in that part of the gaol at Newgate known as the Pit. In a letter to the town sheriff he attacked the confinement of seventeen men in a vault eight feet high and fourteen feet square. As there was no light and no ventilation he was surprised, he said, that they did not all die of suffocation.

Similar concern over the containment of the insane soon followed, inspired by the French Revolution, during which he continued his disreputable links with England's hostile neighbour. On one visit he is thought to have contacted Philippe Pinel, a giant in the history of psychiatry who had persuaded Robespierre and company to apply the new *liberté* to his Paris madhouse. Not only did the unrestrained inmates show no inclination to rampage through the streets as most people had predicted but in many cases their sanity improved. Fox was impressed and in 1794 took over a Quaker asylum at Cleeve Hill, to the north of Bristol, to copy Pinel's example. In 1804, he built Brislington House.

Rather than tie up his patients or allow them to rot in bed, Fox encouraged them to take the air in the leafy hospital gardens, which he made more peaceful by the release of pheasants and doves. Other treatments supplemented the congenial milieu. In deference to nearby Bath, Fox made balneology a feature of his care but more influential still was his belief in animal magnetism.

This curious therapy had little to do with magnetism and nothing at all to do with animals, except, as will become clear, in the case of Edward Fox. It was essentially a cross between hypnosis and touching and was closely connected with the name and reputation of Anton Mesmer. Believing (probably) that nervous illnesses arose from an imbalance in the 'magnetism' which permeated the human body and the atmosphere, Mesmer designed a treatment to set the deviant forces straight. Based on a contraption called a baquet – a barrel full of bottled magnetic water with protruding iron bars – the treatment required patients to hold on either to the bars or each other.

After claiming dramatic success, Mesmer was drummed out of his native Austria as a charlatan and so settled in Paris, where animal magnetism was quickly the object of suspicion. In 1784 Mesmer's exploits were scrutinized by a Royal Commission headed by Benjamin

Franklin, the US ambassador to France. Distinguished scientists were recruited to study the phenomenon, including the chemist Lavoisier, who had named both hydrogen and oxygen, and the physician Guillotin whose own contraption would within a decade cut short the exploits of countless more men, including Lavoisier. The commission came down heavily against Mesmer. Franklin summed up its view by saying, 'Imagination is everything, magnetism nothing.'

None of this dampened Edward Long Fox's interest. Perhaps he was attracted to the physical comfort which remained once animal magnetism was stripped of its wilder rituals. Yet he also had faith in hypnosis and so, soon, did his many patients. For any who doubted, he could produce a compelling argument: a bull he had entranced, on whose back he would ride around the same countryside where I was now driving.

Unlike his friend Beddoes, Fox lived into his seventies, the best known alienist of his day. And he might have been better known still because in 1811 he was summoned to Windsor to attend George III, who was suffering another flare-up of the madness nowadays attributed to porphyria. Fox made the journey east but could not be persuaded to become the King's physician. Apparently his republican sympathies and his liking for notoriety were as strong as ever.

I had imagined the spa water drunk in the Bath Pump Room to be pungent and powerful, the sort of thing Dr Jekyll quaffed en route to Mr Hyde but the liquid I was offered when I arrived there could barely emit a single blast of sulphur. Sensing my let-down, the waiter assured me it was just as putrid as ever, despite the filtering out of clay which now precedes its sale. I took a swig. It was insipid rather than foul, an unwise choice for a potion with medicinal pretentions.

Around 1670 the young Daniel Defoe must have been one of the first to swallow the stuff, yet he was surprised to find that drinking it had become fashionable when he returned to Bath fifty years later. John Radcliffe, the doctor whose name is on two Oxford hospitals, is supposed to have been responsible for the change although Defoe didn't believe that story, his own first taste having occurred too many years before Radcliffe's prime.

Radcliffe has also been credited with introducing Bath to its most celebrated bon viveur, Beau Nash, not out of good will to the town or the man, but out of spite. How the people of Bath insulted the famous physician isn't clear but insult him they must have. Why else would such a distinguished figure have taken the trouble to sabotage their spa by releasing a toad into its murky water? Enter Nash, a gambler and a fantasist, ready to put both roles to good use. He had heard, or so he said, of a Frenchman who, having been bitten by a tarantula, was cured by music. Perhaps toads were equally sensitive. He proposed an exorcism and even played the gentle sounds himself on the fiddle. The toad was never seen again, which certainly was not true of Nash. He had learned that ceremony was all that mattered, whether in the spa or in the town outside.

Glancing up from the counter where the healing brew was being served, I caught the eye of Nash's statue looking back over the remnants of polite society whose rules he once invented. One was a ban on tobacco, others prohibited swords and swearing where ladies were present. For years Nash lorded it over the English gentry as only outsiders are allowed to do. Overdressed and eventually penniless in the best tradition of socialites, he more than anyone made Bath a haven for aristocrats. Yet at the same time he diverted the town's funds towards the treatment of sick paupers.

The Pump Room sculpture catches Nash in the later part of his life, when his portraits made him look shame-faced and flabby, as if caught with his finger in the blancmange. But in the posture of the statue gazing down on the crowds there was also something disapproving, as well there might be. The decorum Nash fostered was a full-blooded pomp, properly powdered and perfumed, while the modern Pump Room, from its gawkish waitresses to its polished aspidistras, is a model of bruised gentility. This is England at its least insightful, unaware of the sniggers it attracts. At the table next to where I now sat to take tea, a group of teenagers from New York had tossed their baseball caps on the tablecloth and were enjoying the show of English manners as if watching a dog doing tricks. By the time I had seen a few more diners cautiously sniffing the spa water they had just ordered, I had had enough and went looking for the unfiltered variety among the Roman ruins.

The water in the baths steams like a swamp, its opaque green hue adding to the impression that it is a leftover of the primordial soup in which life began. Its effect on the visiting hordes is compulsive, more so because a sign warns not to touch it. Everyone dips a hand in, then looks thrilled that it comes out with its skin intact. It is the same spirit that for centuries has led people to plunge in and feel better for it.

A plaque on the wall beside the Great Bath gives a potted account of the spa's discovery but misses the detail that the first patients were pigs. King Bladud was the man responsible for the find, though not until he had become, like his son Lear, a victim of inter-generational conflict. While still a young man, he journeyed to Athens to acquire an education but, legend has it, picked up leprosy as well. On returning to the court of his father Lud Hudibras, he was instantly banished, so much fear did the disease arouse, and so became a swineherd in Swanswick, in the valley of the Avon.

One day as he was driving his pigs around Beechen Cliff, they changed colour, disappearing one by one over the brow of a hill and returning covered in steaming black mud. When the mud dried and fell off, they had been transformed in another way. Until then they had been a blistered, mangy lot but the mud had cured them. Bladud threw himself in the filthy bog and he too came out cured, ready to head back to court and claim his throne. One of his first acts as king was to build a cistern and a city for the soothing waters.

By the time the wall plaque was erected in 1699, spas were in vogue. Water itself had never gone out of fashion, finding its place in pagan ritual, Roman hedonism and Christian anointing. The King's Bath, dedicated to Henry I, was added to the Roman Grand Bath by John de Villula, a Norman physician with a belief in thermal healing – the temperature of the spring is constantly between 114 and 120 degrees Fahrenheit – who later became Bishop of Wells. The Queen's Bath did not follow until Queen Anne, consort to James I, visited Bath in 1616 in the hope of curing her dropsy. She was about to be immersed in the King's Bath when a trick of light on the green water frightened her so much that a new bath had to be constructed for her use.

Ill paupers too travelled to the spa, encouraged by their local parishes, who would otherwise have been obliged to care for them.

Bathing and douching became common treatments for rheumatism, lumbago and neuralgia, although some experts warned that douching would simply drive pains to another part of the body. The hot spring water was also thought to benefit psoriasis and even leprosy, though this may be only a confusion of medical terms as cases of psoriasis were sometimes loosely called leprosy (perhaps one such case was Bladud himself).

James II and his wife Mary of Modena took the waters for another reason: to produce a Catholic heir to the throne. To this end Mary spent weeks in Bath although James was too busy with affairs of state to leave London for more than a few days. That proved to be enough. Mary became pregnant with James Stuart, the father of Bonnie Prince Charlie. But the birthday celebrations did not last long. The King's daughter, also called Mary, and her husband William of Orange, on hearing the news that the throne they were expecting was lost, invaded and drove the Stuarts out of the country. They may have regretted the move because, as I had been reminded in Dorset, they both caught smallpox here a few years later.

Bath became a meeting place for the rich during the reign of Mary's sister Queen Anne, though her initial reason for going there in 1702 was medical. Her husband, Prince George, suffered from gout, dropsy and asthma – he was said to be so breathless, he was lucky to survive the journey there – and all three conditions were treatable with Bath water. Another story, however, makes infertility Anne's reason for taking him there.

Within a few years the tea-rooms were full of the nation's nobility. The attraction may have been something to do with a reputed rise in gout after Portuguese port became popular. More likely it reflected the power of fashion and the wit of Beau Nash. Daniel Defoe was in no doubt that Bath was 'a resort of the sound rather than the sick' and he wrote ironically of the bathing ceremony:

> In the morning you (supposing you to be a young lady) are fetched in a close chair, dressed in your bathing clothes, that is, stripped to the smock, to the Cross-Bath. There the music plays you into the bath and the women that tend you present you with a little floating wooden dish, like a basin; in which the lady puts a handkerchief, and a nosegay, of late the snuff-box is

added, and some patches; though the bath occasioning a little perspiration, the patches do not stick so kindly as they should.

Men and women were supposed to keep to their own sides but, said Defoe, they merely pretended: 'They converse freely, and talk, rally, make vows, and sometimes love; and having amused themselves an hour, or two, they call their chairs and return to their lodgings.'

Nevertheless Defoe was convinced of the medicinal power of the waters, whether bathed in or drunk, 'especially in colics, ill digestion, and scorbutic distempers'. Eminent medical men agreed that relief was possible, not just in cases of pain but in paralysis, chorea, scrofula, and even alcoholism; the warm liquid was the ideal balm for the coldness and anxiety that could turn men to strong liquor.

Eighteenth-century Bath was not simply a health farm for the idle rich. Like its Master of Ceremonies Nash, however much it came to represent frippery, it also had a serious medical purpose. Nash, before he frittered away his wealth, devoted some of it to a hospital to treat the poor and after a short walk from the Roman Baths I came across the legacy of that venture, the National Hospital for Rheumatic Diseases. It had opened as the Royal Mineral Water Hospital in 1739 and bathing and heat have remained part of the conventional treatment of arthritis.

William Oliver founded the hospital to treat gout (he also suffered from it) and similar inflammations of the joints, with spa water. Not only was he a fervent advocate of cure by water, he also, as medical men tend to, applied a strict list of unproven rules to its use and thus cornered the market. The water could not be too hot, or lain in for too long. Bathing was not to be followed by exposure to cold air or an over-hot bed. Anyone who drank inflamed liquor or ate seasoned meats risked death. Instead his patients could eat his own 'nutritious and easily digested food for rheumatic sufferers', the Bath Oliver. For doctors of the age, perhaps of all ages, the proof of greatness was to be remembered in the name of an illness, such as Addison's disease or Sydenham's chorea. Poor Dr Oliver, preserved only as a biscuit.

Alexander Pope described Oliver as 'the freest, the humblest, most entertaining creature you ever met' but, as a governor of the infirmary in Bath, he must despite his virtue have played a part in a notorious medical row in which the pen of Tobias Smollett was also active. It concerned Archibald Cleland who, with Pope's backing, obtained a post at the city's general hospital in 1742, although by then he had already been in conflict with leading local doctors about his offer – which they refused – to use his own money to renovate the spa.

Within a year of Cleland's appointment accusations were flying of a sort that a modern tabloid would relish. Two women, Mary Hudson and Mary Hook, charged him with indecently assaulting them, using the surgical instruments he was in the habit of inventing. They and a witness called Sarah Appleby told a story of locked surgery doors and repeated vaginal examinations. Cleland at first claimed he had been palpating Hudson's uterus; nothing wrong with that as she was, he said, a hysteric and by standard medical lore was likely to be malfunctioning in that region of her anatomy.

As the case, heard by the hospital authorities, began to go against the doctor, mutual hostility grew. The governors said that Cleland had tried to bribe the witnesses. He retorted that the women were whores. There could be only one outcome: Cleland was sacked. After the judgement one of the governors offered physicians everywhere a piece of advice. If he were a doctor, he said, he would never examine a lady 'above the shoestrings or below the necklace'.

But that was not the end. Cleland spent years writing pamphlets of protest, aided by Dr Smollett who, it was uncharitably said, had also failed to break into respectable medical practice in Bath. Smollett lambasted corruption among local doctors which, he was sure, Cleland had been about to expose, hence his dismissal. Furthermore, he identified one William Warburton as the instigator of the case against Cleland. Warburton, Smollett let it be known, had been trying to curry favour with one of the hospital's governors who despised Cleland, in the hope of advancing his plan to marry the governor's niece.

But the closed doors of medical power proved hard to dent. Right or wrong, Cleland remained in private practice and as a doctor Smollett never achieved the fame he managed as a writer. Warburton, on the other hand, was appointed Bishop of Gloucester.

And William Oliver? After he died, his methods went on thriving.

But his therapeutic biscuit could have disappeared with him if he had not entrusted his manservant Atkins with the secret recipe. Atkins was under no illusion about the true value of the Oliver to the people who visited Bath. He opened a shop and made his fortune selling it.

THREE

The valleys of South Wales

Nowhere is as black as a mine shaft with the lights out. Miners compare the darkness to being blind but the mine shaft is more than black – which in any case is not what many blind people experience. It is also oppressive, a blanket that hugs your skin so tightly that no part of you is left visible.

At one time pit ponies lived so long in this darkness that they are supposed to have lost their sight completely, although miners who remember the animals strolling at the pit surface during the summer shutdowns doubt it. 'Not totally blind,' they say, any more than the men themselves became *totally* blind.

In the human case the lack of light has been blamed for miner's nystagmus, an involuntary jerking of the eyeball. The theory is that constant darkness prevents the retina from relaying precise vision to the brain. Vague images are then all that can be formed and the eye responds by jerking just as it does when trying to focus the blur of a moving train. In the 1930s and 1940s there were up to two thousand cases of nystagmus every year but in these days of strip lighting it is almost unknown. Nevertheless the most learned of neurology textbooks, known as 'Little Brain' after its original creator Lord Brain, is sceptical. 'Neurosis,' it says, 'may play a part in maintaining the disorder.' I don't suppose its current author ever stood in a mine shaft.

But there I was in orange overalls, boots, donkey-jacket and helmet, a lamp battery and an emergency oxygen supply strapped to my waist, feeling faintly ridiculous – did I say faintly? – like a new boy at school about to be shown the ropes and the rituals. There I stood in a cage moving at ten metres per second down a 600 metre hole in the ground, also known as the Taff Merthyr colliery. I could see water running

39

down the sides of the shaft. And I could see Bob and Lyn, one the safety boss, the other a nurse, who were there to lead me round and out again in one piece, approximately.

The jokes about death and danger that miners are fond of show how serious a subject safety is. My watch was removed in case the battery sparked an explosion. I would get it back, I was told, if I was alive to use it. Over and over again, the same joke.

I quickly found there is no such thing as a face-to-face conversation down a mine because whenever someone talked directly to me, the light on his helmet was so dazzling that I could not see his face. This had the eerie effect of making voices come from disembodied torches. With Bob there was no chance of a tête-à-tête for another reason. As soon as the cage hit the bottom, he stormed along the main tunnel singing at top volume and once in a while tossing a frightening fact in my direction.

The tunnel was wide and windy, its floor covered with what looked like moon dust. The wind too seemed to come from some flat lunar landscape where nothing could interrupt it or the continuous spray of coal dust it blasted into my eyes and mouth. The stronger the wind, the better the ventilation, Bob stopped singing to tell me. We had reached a huge wooden gate that blocked the tunnel and was impossible to open. Bob pulled a smaller door to equalize the pressure on either side and the gate was now ready to move, letting us into a chamber the size of a church hall, with another gate at its far end. Ventilation in the mine was by a two-shaft system, air from the surface passing down one shaft, blowing round the tunnel to and from the coal-face and back up the second shaft. The double gates acted as a valve, kept shut by pressure differences which also produced the gale we had been facing.

Two-shaft ventilation is one of several ways of dispelling the gases which have been the greatest threat to health for much of the history of coal-mining. Four hundred years ago, the main hazards were black-damp (carbon dioxide), chokedamp (nitrogen) and styth (a cocktail of gases), and the main method of dispersal was to beat the air with a jacket. But in the deeper pits dug in the seventeenth century, an even greater danger seeped out of the coal-face. Unlike its predecessors, firedamp (methane, ironically the same gas which lowered the suicide rate when it replaced town gas in Britain's ovens) is explosive. The first known ignition occurred under Gateshead in 1621 and, as mining increased, so did the deaths, eventually totalling thousands in each coalfield, although there are no records to show how many thousands.

As coal began to fuel the Industrial Revolution, a solution was sought. Two shafts offered one, furnaces and fans were others. For a time, some mines removed the explosive gas by exploding it. A 'fireman' would crawl along the face with a lighted candle ahead of him on the end of a long pole. When the blast came, he ducked. The seam was then gas-free and work could begin.

The problem should have vanished with the invention of the Davy lamp. Humphry Davy, fresh from poisoning poets in Bristol, turned his genius to the design of a lamp that would light up, but not blow up, in a firedamp leak. But paradoxically, deaths from explosions grew after the lamp entered service in 1815 because miners, or at least mine owners, thought they were going to be safer and dug more deeply into methane-rich seams while bothering less about ventilation.

As the incline increased, the floor grew more uneven and Bob stretched his lead over Lyn and me. Pipes and girders began to appear on every side and sensible walking meant positioning my head in the gulley between metal pipes suspended from the ceiling along the length of the tunnel. But the floor was pocked with holes full of black water and from time to time I had to move sideways between a different two pipes to avoid tripping over. So craggy was the ground in places that coal had to be transported towards the surface by a mono-rail hanging from the roof.

I was now stepping through frequent pools, trying to follow Bob's route exactly, and only once was I headstrong enough to plough through a puddle he had side-stepped. I should have guessed it would be as deep as a canyon; I was straight in it up to the shins. 'That's a big one,' Bob said, without slackening.

Dust gave the air a grey haze as if reality itself had become a little faded and on every surface there was thick powder. Bob explained that stone dust was sprinkled on the ground to dilute the coal dust because the latter was combustible. Like much else in the mines, this simple safety measure was inspired by catastrophe. In 1844 an explosion at

Haswell Colliery in County Durham killed ninety-five men and from the speckled burns on the corpses it was clear that something other than firedamp had ignited. A year later the scientist Michael Faraday, previously an assistant to Davy, reported to the Royal Institute that atmospheric coal dust could itself burn and transmit a local blast throughout a mine.

After what must have been several hundred metres, we reached the coal-face to hear that the tunnel at its other end was 'gassed out', methane having reached the critical level at which men are withdrawn. The seam itself was being worked as usual. The entrance to the face looked like a scrapyard, there were so many chunks of metal to climb over. The pipes that had guided us this far multiplied along the floor and walls, the ground became more ragged and unpredictable and the lighting was left to our own helmets. Although the seam was over 2 metres high the passage beside it was not much more than one metre and varied according to the undulations underfoot. This meant either walking bent double, which was quickly painful, or crawling through pools of mush. What made the discomfort worse was that our route was continually blocked by girders, or equipment, or men squatting beside machines which they were turning on and off.

In the darkness I had no time to realize when I was alongside anything human. The men's blacked-out faces blended with the walls and made their eyes large and mournful, as if they had been plucked from photos taken in 1926. I edged past them, fell against them and stood on them. 'How are you liking it?' they shouted, with more pity than mockery.

It made me think about George Orwell on his pit visit *en route* to Wigan Pier, a lanky sophisticate ogling a subterranean world, likening the men to trolls and admiring their mobility in such a cramped space. They in turn must have marvelled to see him and, to judge by how often they asked how I was liking it, they would have been pleased he found their workplace so unbearable.

It had become too hot to be dressed as I was. My hands were filthy from creeping and steadying myself against anything solid, whether animal or mineral. I didn't try to count how often my helmet thudded against a roof beam. But a brief stop to watch the seam being cut gave me a chance to compare the state of my legs and lungs. Neither was in a winning mood. The next shadow I slumped against was a man who said it didn't matter before I had time to apologize. I knew what he was about to say so I asked him how *he* was liking it. I couldn't understand what his job was but I could see it meant pushing a lever all day. It was OK, he confided, but tedious.

Something was wrong here. I had spoken to a man who spent each working day sitting in darkness a kilometre below the surface of the earth and had discovered only that he was bored. Neither he nor anyone else so much as grumbled about the lack of room. One man went as far as to tell me that even at the smallest seam, there was always plenty of space. This was hard to swallow, except by imagining the mine as part of a vast underground, limitless rather than confined. To those who were stuck down here, it was like the sea and just as spacious. No one on board ship complains of claustrophobia and the same is true of mines.

Once the circular blade had hacked its way past us along the seam, we were up and off again, Bob nimbly manœuvring round objects I couldn't see. In places, the sodden coal dust at our feet was bubbling steadily but no one seemed to worry about the gas. 'It's our very own spa,' someone said, spotting my doubtful expression.

I was now making progress by a painful waddle which had the virtue of being drier than shuffling on all fours. I decided to tell Bob I wanted to head back. I had got the idea: conditions were lousy. But he was too far in front to hear. Then he stopped, because the coal-face had come to an end.

Where we rested the noise of machinery barely reached and the carbon powder in the air seemed to deaden our voices. It was light and the tunnel was broad again, and from our position we could look directly along a spout-hole, the shortest, narrowest route to the top. It was no more than 60 centimetres high and wide but it was the exit for casualties except, as one miner put it, for fat men on stretchers. In A. J. Cronin's autobiographical novel *Adventures in Two Worlds*, which, I suppose, is his life story jazzed up with fantasy, he has to crawl down a tunnel of similar size and amputate a miner's leg. On his first day as colliery doctor, as well. And on his honeymoon.

A pit manager sat with us, testing the air for gas. If there was 1.4 per cent methane, electrical power had to be cut. When it reached 2 per cent, men were removed from the area, though not far. At 10 per cent there was a danger of explosion but at 15 per cent there would be insufficient oxygen to blow up. 'We don't worry about 15 per cent,' said the manager. 'In any case, at that reading we're all unconscious.' This was the area that had been gassed out earlier that morning and it still read 2 per cent. No one else moved so I sat where I was, without knowing much about where that was, except a long way down.

Over the centuries of mining in South Wales there has been a lot more to being unhealthy than can be put down to the invisible, odourless explosive I was inhaling. As soon as digging went below the earth's surface, there was danger, the hills being so waterlogged that men were frequently drowned. One mediaeval wag remarked that the industry gave its handsomest profits to the undertakers. But, as a source of death and disease, coal-mining flourished in the industrial boom of the nineteenth century.

Welsh pits were among those that made children as young as five a key defence against water and firedamp by employing them as 'trappers'. Their task was to open the doors to allow coal wagons through, the same doors that ensured ventilation. If they didn't do that, they worked the water pumps. Either way, their legs spent the day partially immersed in wet filth and consequently were usually swollen and often infected. Worse still was the job of dragging baskets of fresh coal from the seam along passages less than half a metre high. The soon-to-be-Earl of Shaftesbury's commission, investigating child labour, noted that the mortality of children engaged in mining was four or five times what it was in agricultural areas.

The impact of Shaftesbury's report, submitted to Parliament in 1842, was intensified by drawings of women and children labouring under the ground. One member of the commission, a doctor called Southwood Smith, made the tart remark that MPs who believed they were too busy to read the facts could look at the pictures, and his cynicism about government concern was to some extent borne out. Not for the last time, Westminster was in cahoots with the mine-owners, who were keen to go on paying children a sixth of what they paid adult men. When the Mines and Collieries Act emerged, its most radical proposals had been blunted.

Nevertheless it was no longer legal to employ children under ten underground and female labour was prohibited. Only recently, when it became anti-egalitarian to ban women from the coal face, were they given the right to return to the pits. Lyn was amused by the prospect. 'We haven't had any women applying yet,' he shrugged.

It proved too difficult for Shaftesbury to stick to his brief and comment only on the working conditions of children. He also listed some of the diseases older miners suffered. Many of them affected the lungs but heart disease was also commonplace, as was every kind of gut-rot, a result of relieving thirst with mine water. Rheumatic complaints too were abundant. A hundred years later Orwell also referred to bent spines and callouses between the shoulder-blades caused by multiple collisions with the low roof beams.

Yet by mid-century, a third of all deaths in the mines were from respiratory disorders, as many as from injury. Most notorious was the black spit, the result of breathing fine coal fragments, a cause of weakness, breathlessness and death. Laboured breathing could also be a sign of miner's asthma, particularly in young men. And most miners were young, their average age of death in the 1850s being twenty-seven.

Both miner's asthma and black spit seemed to diminish in the second half of the nineteenth century and mortality rates were quartered as safety and air were both forced by law to improve. But the same symptoms reappeared under a new name after the Great War: coalminer's pneumoconiosis, the most infamous of all occupational diseases, especially in South Wales where it was forty times more common than in the rest of the country's collieries.

Progress was to blame. As coal-face machinery grew better at cutting seams, it also grew better at pulverizing them, filling the air with a delicate and easily-inhaled coal dust. Part of the fault, though, lay with complacency, arising from a piece of medical folklore concerning an immunity the dust was believed to confer.

With folklore you win some and lose some. Edward Jenner had listened to a milkmaid in Old Sodbury and made one of the greatest medical discoveries. But thousands of Welsh miners were victims of a belief held by doctors and bosses that coal dust was not only harmless but actually prevented tuberculosis. The lopsided logic went like this: the silicosis of stone dust was by definition a fibrotic lung disease which predisposed to TB; TB was uncommon among miners; so coal, unlike rock, did not cause fibrosis of the lungs. But it did, as the thousands of disabled cases in the 1930s and 1940s proved. It was more likely that the low rate of TB in coal workers had another explanation: gullible doctors, expecting not to find it and coming up with the wrong diagnosis.

The particles of dust which give rise to pneumoconiosis are of a specific size, between one half and seven millionths of a metre, small enough to reach the deepest recesses of the lungs and big enough to block their lymphatic drainage system when they get there. The most virulent variety comes from anthracite because of its 'high rank', a term applied to coal of high carbon content. This may account for the colossal amounts of disease in the Welsh valleys, which are rich in high rank coal. It may also be down to bad luck. Welsh mines were quick to be mechanized and so were first to witness the explosion in lung fibrosis.

By 1929 the South Wales Miners' Federation had won their campaign for a compensation scheme for men whose lungs had been damaged by exposure to coal dust alone. Previously miners had had to prove that they had worked in an environment where stone dust, the cause of silicosis, was also present because coal dust was still viewed as benign. But when the toxicity of coal became obvious, the rules for compensation relaxed a little and claims increased. In 1945, the peak year for claims in South Wales, 5,000 cases were accepted as showing partial or total disability but even this figure was only 60 per cent of those who thought themselves affected. In the worst mines that year, one in three underground workers was certified as having the disease.

The compensation panel was never renowned for being generous but its excuse was medically sound, if overplayed. The natural history of pneumoconiosis is not natural. It can be clearly present on X-ray without producing any symptoms and leads to breathlessness only when the lungs are heavily shadowed. What makes compensation still harder to judge is that miners have often smoked tobacco. Cigarettes and coal dust seem to add to each other's risk of causing both pneumoconiosis and bronchitis. So when a smoker with mild fibrosis on X-ray is breathless, it is judged to be because of his bronchitis and he may not receive any money. But because the bronchitis could have been less severe if it were not for the dust, refusal may be unjust. Miners used to feel – still do – that no one was ever given more than he deserved.

The unusual discrepancy between disability and what shows up on film has been behind a successful screening programme of regular X-rays which detects symptomless cases and transfers them to a less polluted workplace. That is one reason why there were 4,000 new cases of 'pneumo' in Britain in 1950 and only 400 in the mid-1980s. Another is that there is less dust to breathe; one miner told me that in the 1950s the dust was so thick when the cutters were running that you could not see beyond arm's length. A third reason is that most of the pits are now closed. Even so, the drop in incidence is real. Whereas thirty years ago one in seven coal-workers was affected, the rate had fallen to less than 2 per cent by 1983. In South Wales it was still three times the national figure.

Lyn saw it as a disease of the past and knew only two men at Taff Merthyr who were certified, Bob being one. Lyn's main task was dressing injuries to hands and eyes. 'They're a tough bunch. They call in at the end of a shift and say, "I've chopped my finger off. Put a plaster on it, will you?"' More miners' humour, I supposed.

We were walking back through the main tunnel now. The return trip along the coal-face had been less eventful, as return trips tend to be. In Bob's singing there was no sign of the one other sickness I had heard was rife throughout the coal fields: loss of morale, the product of an industry in disarray. In the 1950s, when the older miners of Taff Merthyr first pulled on their donkey-jackets, there were 200 working pits in South Wales. At the time of my visit there were five.

It is a final insult, the latest in a long line. Coal-mining may have created a coherent purpose in the towns of the Welsh valleys but it has also exploited their dependence on it. It has drowned their men, scarred their lungs, gassed, burned and crushed them. When it suited the industry, men had their wages cut, as in 1926, or were thrown out of work. In 1931 61 per cent of Merthyr men were jobless. Faced with such outrage, it would be hard to disagree with the miner-poet Idris Davies at his anguished best:

> O what is man that coal should be so careless of him,
> And what is coal that so much blood should be upon it?

It was Davies's view that coal was not worth all the trouble and I was ready to agree. It is almost compulsory in liberal circles to worship the coal industry and believe in its survival, and for laudable, liberal reasons. But I left Taff Merthyr thinking the mines were a foul place to work and could not be depopulated too quickly. Of course there are counter-arguments about employment and communities, about the dignity of miners and their labour. But the dignity of mining and its people is a pride which has grown out of suffering. It would not exist without the indignity of ill health and injury, to which it is a reaction just as the morbid wit is a reaction to the danger.

Coal-mining is doomed, there can be no doubt about that. In fifty years it will seem like slavery, a vulgar facet of an unenlightened time. This is less than those who have cut the coal deserve but then they have always deserved better.

It was a sentimental plan, to take the Heads of the Valleys Road east and loop into Ebbw Vale and Tredegar, the home ground of Aneurin Bevan, but too compelling an idea to resist. In the late 1940s Bevan bludgeoned and bribed the medical profession into accepting the National Health Service and now personified its founding principles. I was intrigued to see where his own principles had been born.

Although Bevan did not invent the NHS, he still looks like its true progenitor. From his early career in the miners' unions he was in a good position to witness the link between poverty and ill health, and to see the advantages of a health care system that was 'free at the point of use', a phrase that has assumed the status of a commandment. The more extreme critics at the time when Bevan was Minister of Health and Housing warned that a free health service would be exploited by malingerers but this has not been a problem. Its real difficulty has been in coping with the extent of genuine need.

The National Health Service has presided over immunization, cancer screening, antenatal care, microsurgery, and the successful treatment of heart disease and mental illness. Yet one of the most striking achievements of Bevan's creation has been the change in attitudes that it has produced, as important to its future survival as any of its more measurable benefits. Free basic health care has come to be seen in Britain not as an ideal but as a right, more so than homes and jobs, which are similarly affected by poverty.

Nowhere has this change been more remarkable than in the medical profession, many of whose members opposed the Health Service at its inception. Doctors were once suspicious of Bevan's intentions. Now they are fiercely protective of his original purpose and suspicious instead of the administrative changes that successive governments have introduced, fearing that they could undermine the purpose of the NHS: the equal treatment of patients based on need rather than demand. One of the most enduring effects of what was done in 1948 when the Health Service came into being has been the irreversible conversion of the people who work in it.

Illuminating though Michael Foot's biography of Bevan is, it says little about his earliest childhood or the street where he grew up. There is something enticing in a person's earliest home and the ordinary things he did there, something which can never be found anywhere he frequented once his name was made. To the visitor years later, there can be an impression of looking in on destiny, however pompous that may at the same time feel. The thought always appears: when he was here, he did not know what was coming. When Aneurin Bevan lived in Charles Street, Tredegar, he did not know where he would end up, but of the spirit that would dominate the House of Commons and the conference hall, more might be revealed in Charles Street than in any scene of his adult triumphs.

I was quickly in the centre of Ebbw Vale, which is not far from the rest of Ebbw Vale, the town where Bevan was MP for thirty years. The centre is one building, not a church or even a colliery, but a multistorey car park. Turning up a hill to the right I decided to stop and look over this part of the valley.

A side-street among terraced houses seemed to be offering the sort of panorama which I imagined would reveal the romantic essence of the valleys; I turned into it and inched forward. The first road block was a crowd of children too young even to have been forced down the pits in the last century, one carelessly assaulting the others with a skipping rope. Although they moved slowly and reluctantly, the street in front of me cleared after a few minutes, the infants conducting their beatings on the pavement.

The second road block was a football match and the teenage players glared at my intrusion. I braked and got out. To my surprise the town had disappeared in a mist that must have settled as soon as I stepped outside to look. The footballers watched sullenly for a moment, then turned away without interest. In an unmarked building ten metres away a bingo caller completed the scene.

I didn't stay long before retracing my route past the infant crowd, one of whom was standing at the kerb as I approached. I slowed down. She peered in at me with deep round eyes that resembled the eyes of a miner blacked up with coal dust and, still on the look-out for romance, I imagined generations of hardship in her expression. A sudden thud jolted the car. The girl held up a huge stick and didn't blink.

Tredegar was under a similar haze as I descended Georgetown Hill, a parody of the dust cloud it must have sported when the local mines were in full swing. I had climbed out of Ebbw Vale and over a rough hill whose bumps and craters made it seem to be struggling to hold in its innards. As late as when Bevan was a local politician, it was said that each valley was distinct from its neighbours but it was hard to see how this town differed from where I had just left, except that Tredegar was more obviously crouched round its snake of a main road.

If I had not bought a map I would not have been able to find Charles Street, though it formed a section of the central route that wound along a line of shops, churches and housing estates. None of the streets wore a name-plate, as if no one who did not already live there would ever want to visit.

Bevan was born in number 32 and lived in number 7 until he was an adult. A large part of the street has since been knocked down and reconstructed, other parts have simply been knocked down. Number 7 is a patch of waste ground, 32 is an overgrown field, and adjacent to it stands a row of bulky houses in suburban style, trying to be distinguished with the help of names rather than numbers. There is nothing at all to recall the founder of the National Health Service.

My map showed there was a Bevan Avenue nearby which, although I had given up hope of any worthwhile discovery, I could not leave without seeing. It too had no name-plate. The streets of the surrounding estate were identical to those in any other industrial town in Scotland or the North-east: the same beige houses with grimy eaves, the same gardens growing only nettles, the same satellite dishes, the same teenagers driving too fast in old Ford Escorts. Bevan Avenue – I liked the 'avenue' – was a miserable spot and it was amazing that the people clustering in it did not look equally miserable.

I had not expected much and I had been right. After all, that is the pattern, even the point, of sentimental journeys; they taste sweet with disappointment. Walking to the car, I passed a school above Charles Street. It was too modern to have been the young Aneurin's school where he first stood up for disadvantage. When his teacher mocked a boy who blamed his absence the previous day on the fact that his brother was wearing the shoes, the eight-year-old Bevan threw his ink-well at the man in disgust. Apart from the school, there was nothing else in the street, other than a shoe shop.

On leaving school at the age of fourteen, Bevan went down the mines. But when he became politically active with the South Wales Miners' Federation the colliery owners used his nystagmus as an excuse for not continuing his employment. The industry was then at a peak but Bevan himself wrote, 'When the pit dies, the village dies too; when the pit is ill, the village groans. Each is interwoven with the life of the other.'

The pits have mostly died since Bevan was in one and the towns are decayed. Their heroes, it seems, are heroes only in other places.

FOUR

Bolton

J. B. PRIESTLEY didn't think much of where I was now driving. 'Between Manchester and Bolton,' he wrote, 'the ugliness is so complete that it is almost exhilarating. It challenges you to live there.'

Perhaps that is why the road into Bolton from the south-east has been constructed in a way that for most of the route conceals what you are driving through. From the main highway it is hard to see much of the landcape that lies less than a stone's throw away and the ugliness is only hinted at through empty billboards and garage forecourts with their pumps uprooted. I wondered whether I would see Bolton in the distance, smoking on a flat horizon, but it appeared only for a few moments, with its factory chimneys extinguished, before I arrived in its middle.

The northern industrial town has proved a reliable source of inspiration to artists since it reared its ugly, choking head in the late eighteenth century and their impression of degraded humanity feeding a vast and punishing mechanical overlord has stuck. Dickens was reputedly writing about Preston when he invented Coketown, the setting for *Hard Times*, though he could equally have been portraying half a dozen other places in Lancashire:

> It was a town of red brick, or of brick that would have been red if the smoke and ashes had allowed it; but, as matters stood it was a town of unnatural red and black like the painted face of a savage. It was a town of machinery and tall chimneys, out of which interminable serpents of smoke trailed themselves for ever and ever, and never got uncoiled.

Dickens described it, Lowry painted it and so sharp was their vision of the way towns like Preston and Salford once looked that the image has persisted. Although it was an artistic impression and should have been ephemeral, it has survived by becoming confused with a caricature of the North and its blunt, pigeon-fancying inhabitants which is now so crudely out of date as to be ludicrous, laughable to the people who live there, and kept alive only by a handful of stand-up comedians and local politicians desperate for national recognition. On the once-cobbled streets of Bolton, it is today mirrored sunglasses rather than cloth caps that predominate. It may not be a fashionable town but it still has its fashions and these, as in most of Britain, have more in common with Brooklyn than with Coketown.

Like the old chimney towers now scattered among the housing estates, the town hall must in Victorian England have signalled the power of the provincial borough. Both were edifices of the new industrial age, built higher than anything the area had seen before. In the first half of the nineteenth century Bolton, already a textile town, became the centre of the cotton industry, thriving on the new machines invented by Lancashire men to make the processing of cotton more efficient. People poured into its dilapidated houses to take advantage of the available work and in the fifty years from 1800 the population multiplied from 17,000 to 61,000. So dependent on cotton did Bolton become that when the American Civil War caused the supply of raw crop to dry up the inhabitants starved.

Today the town hall borders a shopping precinct that stands where there was once a collection of pubs and slums. As Bolton grew prosperous, its expanding population became ill from overcrowding and unhealthy working conditions; cotton, while turning it into a boom town, inflicted its own diseases. I wanted to see what remained of Bolton's sickly past and I parked near a bus garage and set off on foot. From the kerb an old man the worse for drink and probably mentally ill was yelling indiscriminately. A smiling policeman, looking on, gave me a reassuring flick of his head. 'Just shouting,' he said.

Across the road from where the buses stop is a crescent of buildings that seem to have been modelled on Georgian Bath, an attempt perhaps to give the town a natural grandeur, always the envy of the *nouveau riche*. Now the crescent acts as a border between two local council worlds. On the bus garage side the doors in the building open into housing offices, on the other side they lead into libraries and look over the shoulder of the town hall at a piazza that has been built on a European model. I stepped through an arch from one scene to the other, from the world of benefit payments to the world of local culture. At one end of the square a religious rock band and their leaflet-carrying entourage were yodelling through a distorting amplifier, turning the heads of passers-by and quickly accosting those who dropped their pace. It made me wonder about the potential power of the Church if it ever mastered the use of the microphone.

With its broad stairway and pillared facade the town hall likewise is turned up too loud and when I strayed inside it seemed that everything was named after Prince Albert, adding to the feeling that someone had overdone the classical pretensions. But it is a people's palace, populist in philosophy and hospitable to its citizens. I followed some other intruders around its corridors to discover what they were making for and found myself facing a hall of aerobics enthusiasts. The Victorian mayors would have choked at the sight.

The period that the town hall celebrates was a thriving one for the town's economy but miserable for its health. In 1848 a man called John Entwisle, of whom little is otherwise known, wrote to the mayor, Thomas Ridgway Bridson, a 'Report of the Sanatory Condition of the Borough of Bolton'. In it he disputed some recent findings by Edwin Chadwick, the eminent reformer of London's sanitation, on the mortality of the town's population but disputed them in a way that made them more emphatic. Chadwick had calculated the average age at death of three classes of Bolton society. Gentlemen, 'persons engaged in professions' and their families, could expect to live on average until they were thirty-four – not much to celebrate unless you compared their prospects to those of tradesmen and their families who died at twenty-three, and to 'operatives' (mechanics, servants and labourers) who with their immediate kin lived on average only to the age of eighteen.

Chadwick had got it wrong, wrote Entwisle, in what must have seemed like irony or at least cold comfort. The true figure for tradesmen was twenty-seven years while for operatives it was nineteen. But he also revealed that these frightening facts disguised the point that in all classes those who survived to their twenty-first birthday lived on average until they were over fifty. The low life expectancy at birth reflected more than anything the terrifying mortality in children under five, who accounted for more than half of all deaths, and in particular in infants under one. In the mid-nineteenth century Bolton's rate of mortality in infancy was about 25 per cent of all live births, and rising.

I left the town hall and cut through the shoppers to reach Deansgate, one of the town's central streets where the risks of urban living at the peak of the Industrial Revolution were once evident. Up alleys that no longer exist whole families would crowd into one room and frequently into one bed. Filth and refuse accumulated and the absence of ventilation allowed the putrid air to linger. Gin, bad food and the lack of light added to the misery and the risk of disease. Entwisle referred to people packed into a room above a slaughter-house. In Gaffer's Ginnel, a back street between Deansgate and Bridge Street at its eastern end, he had seen seventy residents of one building living in squalor beside a tobacco factory and a cesspool. It was these conditions that Entwisle blamed for the higher mortality in towns compared to rural areas because, he informed the mayor, more than one in five deaths resulted from epidemic infections encouraged by the lack of space, sun, nutrition and hygiene.

By 1873, when Bolton produced its first report on public health, the population had increased to around 90,000, ensuring that the over-crowding was as bad as ever and the likelihood of death in infancy just as great. According to John Livy, the Medical Officer of Health for the borough that year, the average age of death for all classes in the town was twenty-two and in some central areas it was only eighteen, suggesting that at best there had been no improvement in survival in the quarter-century since Entwisle's plaintive letter. Livy calculated that 50 per cent of all deaths in 1873 were of children under five and almost a third were less than one.

The main killer was still infection, though in a variety of guises. A quarter of deaths at all ages resulted from 'zymotic diseases', a term suggesting fermentation of some disease-carrying entity as the cause of illness, a theoretical understanding favoured by doctors of the period. The most deadly zymotic diseases were smallpox, measles, scarlet fever, whooping cough, typhus, typhoid, cholera and 'diarrhoea', the last presumably referring to what would now be called infant gastro-enteritis. But in addition diseases of the lungs caused another quarter of the town's deaths and these too were usually infections listed in public health records as bronchitis, pneumonia and phthisis (tuber-culosis). Under the age of one the main risks were from whooping cough and diarrhoea while those who died between one and five were most likely to do so from scarlet fever.

Dr Livy's preoccupation was sewage. When combined with the crushed, overpopulous living space it could be lethal. But in his view it had another, equally damaging effect, because it also kept the poor in their place, limiting their social and spiritual progress. 'The rela-tions of sanitary reform to mental enlightenment are more intimate than at first sight appears,' he wrote in his report. Seeing the restric-ted horizons and the absence of refinement of those who were crammed into back alleys he refused to blame them for their lot. Like a good public health doctor, he accused neither the virus nor the man who coughed it around, saving his powder for the milieu that allowed it to spread so easily. But he went further, suggesting that if the working folk of Bolton were crude, passive and corrupt then that too could be attributed to the filth in which they were expected to live. 'The sanitary improvement of the people is an indispensable pre-liminary to their social elevation and improvement,' he commented. 'Until persons have attained a certain degree of physical comfort in regard to their dwellings and the atmosphere they breathe, it is useless to expect that any of the higher qualities will, to any great extent, take root.' His solution to these woes was a practical one, borrowed from another Lancashire working town, Rochdale. Experi-ence there, he insisted, showed that toilets should be positioned away from actual dwelling space, at a distance from any place where families might congregate. The outside toilet, that late twentieth-century symbol of poverty, officially used by the government as an index of social deprivation, was about to be welcomed as a saviour.

Where I was now walking must once have been a haven for lethal bacteria, probably the only living creatures that could have expected an uninterrupted life-span in nineteenth-century Bolton. Yet epidemics and contagious diseases were not the only problem. Heavy drinking of spirits was a common pastime for adults and children and liver cirrhosis was not unknown to occur before puberty. Even worse, youngsters frequently died of convulsions brought on, according to John Entwisle, by parents who administered gin and opiates in the form of cordials to their offspring.

Entwisle took a dim view of the Rabelaisian scenes on the streets of downtown Bolton in his day and felt strongly enough to give Mayor Bridson the benefit of his opinion on the contemporary notion that working in the cotton mills led women to mature early, an undesirable fate, and to age prematurely. Not so, said Entwisle, because 'it is well known that a low state of public morals has the effect of producing early development'. This moral theme was one he returned to in an article called 'Light upon dark places' in the *Bolton Journal* some thirty-six years later, though it would be wrong to interpret his abiding impression of his fellow citizens as a piece of judgemental Victorian bluster. It is his pity for their dreadful exist-ence that most clearly stands out in an image of industrial Britain that is pure Dickens:

> There are in all large towns certain districts in which all the elements of moral corruption and physical disease and misery acquire an undisputed supremacy where the greatest immorality and the most abject wretch-edness combine to present a picture of human society so utterly revolting that none except the most heroic philanthropist will voluntarily enter them.

Not that the cotton trade, whatever its role in propelling girls into adulthood, had any reason to be complacent. When, thanks to the burgeoning demand for cotton clothes and the ingenuity of men such as Arkwright and Crompton, it ceased to be a cottage industry and moved instead to the factories of innumerable Lancashire towns and waterside locations, it soon had few rivals as a source of occupational disease, mainly related to the dust. In a letter published in 1842 one William Dodd, on a tour of the county, wrote to the Earl of Shaf-tesbury describing the accidents, amputations and pollution of cotton mills, likening their atmosphere to a heavy fall of snow and commenting that the protection of the workers amounted to handkerchiefs worn over their faces.

The illnesses arising from the processing of cotton spanned the life of the industry and were still being commented upon after the Second World War. Over the whole period three principal lung disorders were identified, though their symptoms overlapped, as well as an unusual form of cancer.

Mill fever was a reaction to a person's first exposure to ambient dust; it was not, however, an immediate reaction but a delayed response, starting the night after a first day in the mill. As its colloquial alias – cotton cold – implies, it was a syndrome of cough, dry throat, headache, lethargy and high temperature and the initial attack was short, lasting only a few hours. By the next day it was gone but by the following night, after another day's work, it was back. Yet it was nothing serious, merely a mild, irritating introduction to the dusty air, lasting for several weeks until tolerance developed, although it recurred on a return to the mill after a period away as short as two weeks.

In some ways byssinosis was its mirror image, requiring several years of exposure to cotton or similar fibres. Resembling chronic bronchitis in its appearance, it caused wheezing, coughing and tightness in the chest and in its early stages these symptoms recurred immediately on returning to work, after an absence as short as a weekend, hence its own nickname, Monday fever. But unlike cotton cold it grew worse as time passed, according to one explanation because of a gradually increasing sensitivity to the outer coating of cotton seed. Inevitably raw fibre contains seed fragments in appreciable amounts. If inhaled, so the theory runs, they stimulate cells in the lining of the lung to release chemicals such as histamine, capable of constricting the airways in a sequence of physiological events analogous to those that produce asthma. As exposure continued, Monday fever would slowly affect the whole week and the breathlessness became debilitating enough to put an end to any career in the mills.

A similar deteriorating course awaited those who developed weaver's cough, said to have been the result of handling mildewed yarn and possibly an allergic reaction to one of the many microscopic fungi that grew in it. From the mid-nineteenth century weaver's cough was recognized as a threat to the health of those who worked in carding, stripping and grinding, causing permanent breathlessness and premature death, and it was known as stripper's or grinder's or cotton card-room asthma.

Carding was the process of separating thin threads of cotton from bales into parallel strands which were then twisted into a stronger yarn before being woven into a fabric. In cotton factories it was performed by serrated revolving drums, a long way from the thistles – generic name *carduus* – that were originally used and these carding cylinders and the engines that drove them had to be maintained and restored. Stripping was the name given to the cleaning of teeth on the cylinders while grinding was the process of reshaping and sharpening them. The exposure to dust in these jobs was massive. Respiratory diseases were three times as common in strippers and grinders as they were in cotton workers employed in other activities and their death rate over the age of fifty-five was found in the 1930s to be three times as high. As late as the 1950s it was said that 80 per cent of strippers and grinders suffered from emphysema, the advanced lung disease to which chronic bronchitis leads and the final stage of weaver's cough.

As if these crippling chest conditions were not enough for the men who worked the cotton (the women, less often employed in the most vulnerable occupations, were not so severely affected), the industry also produced its own malignancy, known as mulespinner's cancer. The mule, an eighteenth-century invention of Samuel Crompton, was a hybrid of two types of spindle designed by James Hargreaves and Richard Arkwright and it was a job of the mulespinner to 'piece' or join broken ends of yarn together when they appeared between the spindle and the adjacent roller.

In 1906 a Manchester doctor, S. R. Wilson, noted that mulespinners were prone to cancer of the scrotum, a disease described in chimney sweeps by Dr Percival Pott during the eighteenth century: a famous occasion in medicine as it was the first time a specific malignant tumour had been identified with a particular occupation. In sweeps the carcinogenic substance had appeared to be soot and it was soon widely believed that the bituminous shale oil used in the cotton factories to lubricate machinery was responsible for the cancer that now affected mulespinners.

The atmosphere in the mills was thick with the same oil and identical tumours sometimes appeared elsewhere on the surface of the body. Yet 70 per cent were found on the scrotum and the curious thing was that most of these were on the left side. It did not take long for doctors who knew the industry to work out why: it was all in the technique of piecing. By established practice it was the left hand that was used to reunite the broken strands of yarn, which were reached by leaning over the barrier that surrounded the machinery. This manœuvre pressed the skin around the left groin against the top of the barrier and into contact with the oily overalls that mulespinners wore. The skin in that part of the body was thus in closest contact with the carcinogenic oil.

In the peak period for Britain's cotton imports and exports, the first two decades of this century, the rate of scrotal cancer in men working in the industry was eighteen times what it was in the male population as a whole. A high rate was universal in the factories, the men in the carding rooms carrying seven times the general risk, but in mulespinners the rate was increased thirty-three-fold and by the time they reached the age of sixty-five their likelihood of developing the cancer was over a hundred times greater than that of men in other jobs. One of the putative reasons for the rising risk in older men was the vulnerability of their drier skin but the main explanation was simply that the irritant oil took several years to do the deed. It needed exposure to the mineral oil lasting at least ten years and in most cases much longer before a tumour would appear. The simple conclusion was that any measure that limited contact between the skin and the ubiquitous oil would reduce the rate of cancer, so one preventive innovation was a pair of shorts which were able to act as a barrier between the left side of the scrotum and the sodden overalls. But the key to prophylaxis was the oil itself. Writing about mulespinner's cancer in 1941, Dr E. M. Brockbank charted a fall in its incidence from the mid-1920s, and put the improvement down to safer oil and less splashing. But in retrospect you could say they hardly needed to bother, those public health and occupational physicians who studied and acted to protect the mulespinners, because the withering of the cotton industry and the modernized methods of what was left of it soon achieved what they wanted. Mulespinners and their cancer disappeared together.

Behind the shops and car-parks some of the old red brick buildings of central Bolton, warehouses and other industrial leftovers, were in fragments. But as far as I could tell they were being demolished rather than allowed to collapse. I guessed that the space they left was going to be filled and that the inner layers of the town were going to be reconstructed, because from what I had seen of its innermost workings Bolton was not at all the faded Victorian upstart that places in the North are sometimes accused of being. The centre looked like a village turned prosperous town, with its parish church end on to a street thronged with shoppers and elsewhere its busy library of local life. None of the famed characteristics of the North-west had survived. Only fifty years ago George Orwell in nearby Wigan had woken to the sound of clogs on cobbled streets but now you could transplant this portion of Bolton into Sussex and no one would know the difference, a fact that would disappoint the townsfolk of the Home Counties only slightly less than it would alarm the residents of urban Lancashire.

I pointed the car up Halliwell Road as a detour from my planned route to the South-west. This part of Bolton, just north of the town centre, was one of its most unhealthy districts a century ago and the housing still looked cramped and ancient. Terraced houses and their thin back yards faced each other across narrow alleys dotted with rubbish-bins and children – Indian and Pakistani children because this is one of Bolton's Asian ghettos, older than what I had seen of the Caribbean enclave in St Paul's in Bristol but about as derelict. As recently as twenty years ago the majority of houses in areas like this still had outside toilets and almost half had no bath, and I suppose immigrants were banished there with the idea that any home was better than none. It was Orwell too who thought that the main problem with this kind of housing was not that it was dreadful, although it certainly was and is that, but that there was not enough of it.

Threading in and out of the back lanes I cut a faltering path to a different side of the Asian experience in Britain. The man I had arranged to see was a doctor to his own community, an Indian GP in a predominantly Asian locality. He was looking after the health of his own race, a practice that virtually no other ethnic culture in Britain has emulated. It reflects two features of immigration from the Indian subcontinent that are not found in combination in any other group: the broad social spread of those who settle here and the parallel society that they are therefore able to establish.

It was by now evening and there was no official surgery but patients were being seen just the same. It gave me time to peruse the posters and leaflets stuck to the waiting-room wall. There was a phone number for an Asian women's aid service, advice on how to look after your heart and a sign that read 'Wash your feet often!' From the consulting room came raised voices and a high-frequency wail. A few minutes later Dr Sudhamony Chatterjee emerged smiling.

His health centre stands in Cannon Street, a twisted through-road between two larger thoroughfares of central Bolton's south-west corner. One of these, Deane Road, is lined by shops that, like the surgery, are run by Asians primarily for their own people. Some stores intoxicate you with the aroma of spices, others offer you the latest videos from the Bombay film industry. In some you can buy from untidy piles of household goods, others have careful window displays of huka pipes, Diwali suits and what are called 'fancy goods'.

Almost nine out of every ten patients on Dr Chatterjee's list are originally from India or Pakistan, although some made it to Britain via Uganda; they had lived there until 1972, when Idi Amin abruptly expelled them. About 60 per cent are Gujerati and predominantly Hindu, the remainder being Muslim. Among the older generations, those who came directly from India, there are many who have little knowledge of English.

It used to be said in medical circles that illnesses which had been waning in Britain, particularly tuberculosis and rickets, had resurfaced in Asian immigrants thanks to a mixture of poor climate, bad housing, inadequate nutrition and, in the case of TB, undetected infection at the time of migration. In the fifty years from 1920 the rate of tuberculosis in Bolton, as elsewhere, fell steadily because of improving social conditions and, later, immunization, but it subsequently rose until in the early 1980s it was twice the national rate. The majority of cases were in manual workers and almost half were in the textile industry but these facts were not new. The change occurring in the early 1980s was that two-thirds of cases were now among immigrants, mostly Asian, and the increase in the number of people affected corresponded roughly to the number of cases in this ethnic group.

It was ten years before this, at the beginning of TB's reappearance, that Dr Chatterjee joined a general practice in Bolton. He had come to the UK, he told me, in the mid-1960s from Calcutta where he had been born and educated, graduating as a doctor in 1963. His initial ambition had been to train as an ear, nose and throat surgeon. 'But it didn't work out,' he added quickly before changing the subject.

At that time in Bolton, in the early 1970s, he found a huge amount of TB, mainly of the lungs but also of the lymph glands in the neck (the same scrofula that Thomas Beddoes in Bristol had treated with inhalation) and sometimes of the intestine. A pool of infected individuals, it seemed, had been able to pass on the tubercle bacillus to others in their community who had arrived in Britain too old to be routinely immunized. The transmission had been aided and abetted by overcrowding in homes and wet weather. It was reminiscent of the way in which contagious diseases had spread in Bolton a century earlier and was not a compliment to the hospitality that this country provides for its new citizens.

Rickets too is a disease arising from poor conditions, particularly deficient diet and lack of sunlight. It is a malformation of children's bones which can impair their ability to walk, though it can start before they are born. It results from insufficient calcium or vitamin D; the vitamin is needed to deposit calcium salts in growing bones, where they are the chief mineral. Both these substances are obtained from food but vitamin D is also manufactured in the skin in a chemical process dependent on ultra-violet light. So the theory runs that moving from a hot country like India or Uganda to a wintry one like Britain reduces the habitual supply of sun. Add to this a preference for staying indoors or being covered with clothes to fight the unaccustomed cold and vitamin D production is bound to go down. If the calcium in the diet is also low, which it can be if it does not include cow's milk or if its absorption is obstructed – allegedly some Indian breads can cause this – then rickets becomes a possibility. As with TB, a disease usually resulting from poverty becomes the lot of immigrants.

But since he first settled in Bolton Dr Chatterjee has seen things change. Although their fate in Britain has varied, some Asians have prospered through business and most have escaped the illnesses of the poor. Round his Cannon Street Health Centre the houses were plain and small with boxed-in gardens but they did not give off the gloom of the streets in the north of the town. 'Now it is different,' he told me. 'About 5 per cent of my patients have had TB, mainly the middle aged, and I see very few new cases. And there is no rickets, particularly since good antenatal care became available.'

So what was the medical problem he faced most? Dr Chatterjee paused for a moment and said, 'The common cold.' Medical knowledge, he explained, was limited among his patients and turning to the doctor for minor ailments was automatic. Consequently his practice was overwhelmingly busy. 'If a child sneezes, it is an emergency. Every night there are many call-outs.'

The phone in the office where we were sitting rang on cue and Dr Chatterjee gave me a look that said, 'See what I mean?' as he picked it up. Whoever was calling was out of luck. Their doctor's response came in clipped tones: 'There's no one here. The surgery's closed.' The caller seemed to persist. 'There's no clinic tonight. Ring back tomorrow,' replied Dr Chatterjee sternly, winking at me to let me know he didn't mean it. 'The problem is I'm too available,' he said.

His patients placed a great deal of faith in medicine and expected it to work instantly. 'They like me to give them pills but they prefer injections. But if they are not well again within a few hours they call me back.' The phone rang again. I could see his point.

Part of their faith lay in the fact that they saw in him a man of their own culture but the surprising thing was that this was true of the Muslims as well as the Hindus and the Indians from both Gujerat and East Africa. Despite the hostility between religions and nations in and around India, this doctor from Calcutta was sought by everyone. Speaking Gujerati and Bengali helped, he believed, as did the gifts and appreciative messages on his wall, written in Urdu and reassuring to Pakistanis. 'They have confidence in me because I know their religion so well. They know I respect all their religions to the same extent. In my surgery I'm strict about this. I tell them: I've got no sex and no religion, in here I'm a doctor.'

Working closely for his compatriots had left Dr Chatterjee unswervingly positive about their lives in Britain. Having seen a poster on a bus shelter in Deane Road broadcasting news of what it termed racist murders, I asked about friction with the local whites. It didn't happen, he insisted. Nor did addiction. 'Alcohol and drugs are not a problem in my practice. I have one alcoholic under my care. Once in a while I hear he is drunk and beating people again. He can be rough, he kicks his wife. I go to his house and he's like a mouse. I tell him: don't drink. He doesn't drink. People listen to me. When they can't control patients with mental illness in the local hospital, they ring me. Even when they are not my patients. Even when they are English. I don't know why they do what I say but over the years I have won their trust; perhaps it is a skill that has been given to me by God.'

The success of a parallel culture lies in its determination to remain separate and the danger it has to contend with is that in new generations its barriers begin to leak. Young Asians in Britain are less keen than their parents to do what their culture expects of them and are attracted instead to the different social values of their host society; these, without much oversimplification, boil down to the independence of women. Dr Chatterjee has encountered the problem many times in his clinic.

'The younger people are going to have trouble because they want to copy westerners. The women try to dominate their husbands while the older ones simply accept that their husbands are boss. The marital difficulties I see are all in young couples who want to live as if they are part of a western civilization. Two or three who were planning to divorce have consulted me first. I say: wait. And they go home together to try.

'Sometimes parents bring in their nineteen-year-olds. The father will say, "Doctor, I have a problem daughter. She thinks we treat her as if she is a little girl." I say, "You must remember she is a woman."

Then I speak to the daughter and she says, "My mother and father want to make me work for the family but I want to find my own job. They rebuke me. They act as if I am a child. My father never discusses anything with me. He doesn't see me as an adult." And I tell her, "That is because you are always arguing. He expects you to obey and he feels insulted." She promises to be more respectful.'

I thought of the shouting and weeping I had heard while waiting for the unscheduled evening clinic to end. 'It was about an arranged marriage,' Dr Chatterjee confirmed. 'I have met a few similar disagreements. Sometimes it is the parents who complain that their daughter is planning to marry a boy she has chosen for herself. I tell them, "You have to compromise. If the boy is in your caste or your religion, you should accept him." '

But for all his sympathy and persuasion, Dr Chatterjee's task was impossible. To patch up divisions between a generation of immigrants that has thrived on cohesion and another that sees rewards in what the West can offer is more than can be hoped for. He must have been aware, beneath his optimism, that he and doctors like him would increasingly have to tend to the woes of a culture in transition. Even for the would-be ear surgeon with the power to make people listen, it was a daunting challenge.

FIVE

Sellafield

THE SEA was so brown it looked like a field of mud and it was several minutes after it came into view over the brow of Stoneside Hill before I realized what it was. In the mist the waves seemed to be streaks of driven snow, their apparent motionlessness an optical illusion caused by the undulating moorland road I was on, a single track that rose, fell and twisted on its way to the Cumbria coast.

'Use not recommended', the sign had said where the track left the main road just beyond Duddon Bridge. But I was tiring of the other drivers – not the farmers and their tractors, of which there were only a handful – but the articulated transporters that muscled me out of their way and the men on car-phones who burned me up while I was viewing the mountains. I imagined that, like me, they were heading for the nuclear power station at Sellafield and I preferred to complete the trip without their company.

Driving across the moor after a convoluted journey along the southern border of the Lake District it was impossible not to think that anything placed in such a distant spot must be hoping to keep people away and, by extension, must be up to no good. And certainly when the location was chosen its distance from anywhere and anybody must have counted in its favour. The original Windscale plant was a Ministry of War factory, producing plutonium for the atomic bomb during and after the Second World War. When, during the 1950s, Britain began to see nuclear power as a source of energy the Calder Hall power station was constructed next to Windscale; in fact plutonium production continued after Calder Hall was plugged in to the national grid in 1956. Now the whole site is part of the Sellafield complex – renamed in an attempt to cast off Windscale's notoriety – where the paired activities of power generation and fuel reprocessing take place.

Descending towards the sea I caught my first sight of the cylindrical cooling towers of Calder Hall, half-hidden by the mist and from my vantage point looking smaller and less imposing than popular prejudice would suggest. But as I followed the coast road north what I could see of Sellafield grew in size and complexity. The twin Windscale piles, the towers above the original nuclear reactors, became visible; they were unforgettable from the films I had seen of the occasion in 1957 when one of them caught fire and caused the country's worst nuclear accident.

Before going to Sellafield itself, I took a short side-step into Seascale, the nearest town to the nuclear power station about two miles away, a coastal village of only two thousand people. But it is the centre of one of the most prominent of all contemporary health controversies: that concerning the rate of leukaemia in the children who live there and its relation to the nuclear industry on its doorstep.

Seascale itself is a drab town clumped on the edge of the Irish Sea and, on the day I went there, battered by a stiffening breeze from the west. The fifty metres of water nearest to the beach was pure froth, fermenting out of control in the unrelenting wind. Its streets and houses were plain and subdued but the local paper looked alarmed, its headline 'Killer disease strikes another blow'. But the killer it meant was heart disease, not leukaemia.

For a decade the evidence of an excess of childhood leukaemia around Sellafield has been increasingly emphatic. The disease is a malignancy, or more accurately a group of related malignancies, affecting the bone marrow or the lymphatic system where white blood cells are produced. Most cases occur in adults but in children the risk is proportionately greater because in young people other cancers are relatively rare. Leukaemia is the commonest malignant disease of children and the commonest cause of death of all diseases of childhood after the age of two. Although it is now a highly treatable illness – well over half of cases affecting young people can be cured – the condition and the name itself remain terrifying and any discussion of it acutely emotive.

There is no single cause of leukaemia but some varieties are clearly linked to abnormalities of certain chromosomes, in other words to disruptions of DNA, the chemical of which genetic material is composed. One known source of damage to DNA is radiation and so radioactive chemicals are potential culprits in leukaemia cases, something graphically confirmed by the increased incidence of the disease in survivors of the Hiroshima and Nagasaki atomic bombs.

Leukaemia in Seascale began to arouse suspicion in 1983 when James Cutler, a journalist who was making a television documentary about the Windscale fire, noticed what appeared to be an excess of the disease in the town's children and young adults. As a result Sir Douglas Black, one of Britain's most distinguished physicians, was appointed to head an inquiry into the occurrence of malignant disease in the area among people under twenty-five years of age. Using official health records of cancer cases, the Black Advisory Group in 1984 confirmed that a cluster of leukaemia existed in Seascale.

But any conclusions from these findings – and the report was anxious not to draw any – could be criticised on the grounds that many diseases are not distributed evenly throughout the country and that random variation in incidence would inevitably lead to areas where there are no cases and areas where there are more then expected. Although statistical analysis suggested that the Seascale cluster was highly unlikely to have occurred by chance, this was still possible. Another argument was that the Black Advisory Group had simply confirmed an observation that had to exist in order to invite study; there would never have been a report if the high rate of cases had not been there in the first place. The normal scientific process begins with an idea which is then tested experimentally, the results being used to confirm or refute the original idea. In the Black Report the results were in a sense the starting point and the subsequent findings were no more than a statistical endorsement. They would have carried more impact if someone had theorized that the rate of leukaemia would be high in Seascale before any observations were made. As the report itself conceded, its findings were the basis for further research, not the last word.

Over the next few years the figures were examined more closely, mainly by a member of Sir Douglas Black's inquiry team, Martin

Gardner, a professor of medical statistics. Gardner was able to show a ten-fold increase in leukaemia among children who were born in Seascale but no increase in children not born in Seascale but attending school there. This distinction made it possible that something about Seascale before or shortly after a child's birth made leukaemia more likely.

In 1990 his research group came up with the most dramatic of explanations, in what became known as the Gardner Report. By comparing young people who did or did not develop leukaemia in West Cumbria, they tested for links between the disease and a host of possible contributory factors. The most striking result was that the risk was six times as high in those whose fathers had received one hundred units of radiation in total before conception, according to occupational records. As the average dose of radiation to people outside the nuclear industry is two and a half units per year, this amount is substantial; but it is not thought to affect a person's health even when given in one burst. As the fathers in the study had received the amount over several years, as had about one in ten of the Sellafield workforce, the exposure was well within the assumed limits of safety. But the implication of the study was that this amount of radiation, while leaving general health unaffected, might be capable of damaging the DNA in sperm in such a way that could cause leukaemia some time after conception.

And as if to emphasize the danger, more evidence had appeared a few days before my visit: a re-analysis of the cases studied by Sir Douglas Black but with the advantage of more precise and complete information. There were five confirmed cases of leukaemia in children under the age of fourteen before 1984 and in a village the size of Seascale this rate is thirteen times the rate in the rest of Cumbria. But the study went further and examined what had happened since the Black Report. If the original findings had occurred by chance or had simply confirmed the presence of an unexplained cluster in Seascale, as critics had argued, then you would not expect to find a high rate again over a different period of time. That would be stretching coincidence and credibility too far.

What was found once again was a high rate of cancer in people under twenty-five, accounted for not by leukaemia but by the related condition of lymphoma. Although there were only two cases, the odds against their appearance by chance were one hundred and forty to one. Outside Seascale there was no increased incidence.

It was all this that had led me to ask to meet one of the Sellafield doctors, someone in charge of occupational health at the plant who, because many of the 8,000 employees of British Nuclear Fuels Limited live in the surrounding towns and villages, would also be familiar with the health of the community. And the Sellafield press office, once I had put in writing what I wanted to talk about, had been quick and welcoming. In the nuclear industry good public relations are highly prized, an antidote to popular fears of cancer and disaster.

For this reason the public face of Sellafield is carefully made up with potted plants, a visitors' tour and a gift shop; there you can buy a game called Fission, a kind of ludo in which some of the squares are marked with the chemical symbol for uranium-235, and something with the name 'nuclear tiddlywinks'. And the people I met were overtly enthusiastic about the nuclear industry. I wondered to what extent this was a defensive reaction to the criticisms that were made of it, most of all by the 'environmentalists', a term pronounced with particular disapproval at Sellafield.

I had arranged to meet Shirley Williams who worked there as a press officer. She had agreed to drive me round the site and escort me to the health department. But shortly after we set off a uniformed policeman at the security barrier waved us down; the identification badge I had been given, marked MEDIA VISITOR, was invisible from where he was standing. I held it up and he gave us the all clear.

'Do you have many intruders?', I asked Shirley.

'Not many,' she said.

'Too far away? Even for saboteurs?'

'We're not worried about sabotage. No one knows where the plutonium is kept. Sabotage isn't the point, protesting is the point. Environmentalists.'

I asked her what the environmentalists did.

'They gather outside, which is fine. It's their right. We provide them with a place to protest,' Shirley said. 'And once in a while we see the Greenham Common women, bless them.' I thought: good public relations – undermine the opposition with tolerance.

'Did you check who I am?'

'I certainly didn't,' replied Shirley in a way that made me wonder if someone else did.

'How do you know I'm not going to chain myself to the railings?'

'We don't,' said Shirley cheerfully.

It was only by driving round it that I became aware of the size of Sellafield. It has a series of roads, innumerable square buildings, and a scattering of conspicuous towers and chimneys. Metal ladders and heavy pipes, sometimes in parallel rows, sometimes in repetitive twists, have been laid as a garland around many of these featureless structures. It is a giant concrete and steel metropolis that gives the impression of a vast methodical industry on the move. Although most of them are out of sight, there are in addition to the permanent workforce a few thousand employees contracted to carry out short-term jobs, a total of at least 12,000 people, the population of a small town.

We drove through the untidy sprawl, Shirley explaining what was happening in each location while I nodded and tried to take it all in. The more intriguing buildings seemed to be mostly defunct, 'being de-commissioned' as the industrial vernacular puts it. There were the two Windscale piles, the towers I had seen from the approaching road, the one nearer us being where the fire occurred. The other was being dismantled and half the bulbous cap at its apex had been removed. Shirley told me that any lessons learned from taking this tower to pieces would help when it came to the more awkward task of demolishing its incinerated neighbour. Further on we came to the futuristic sphere that used to feature in every photograph of the power station, the magazine image of the nuclear industry, an experimental prototype of the gas-cooled reactor. Now nicknamed the 'Windscale golf-ball', it looked almost quaint, a fate that often awaits designs that in the 1960s were regarded as space-age. It too was being de-commissioned.

The early reactors, the four steaming funnels of Calder Hall, were of the Magnox type, the word being derived from the magnesium-based compound that encases the uranium fuel. As at any power station, whatever fuel is used, the intention is to generate heat to produce steam and drive a turbine which in turn produces electricity. Newer reactors such as the advanced gas-cooled models carry out this process more efficiently because higher temperatures and pressures are possible and it is only a matter of time before Calder Hall goes the way of other de-commissioned buildings.

But the controversy of what Sellafield does has gradually moved away from the nuclear reactions that take place there towards the reprocessing that is steadily being expanded. Reprocessing is designed to preserve uranium and plutonium from the end products of energy generation and recycle it, using a chemical separation process that also creates an array of radioactive waste substances. All of these have to be disposed of safely. The most toxic are now incorporated in a kind of molten glass, cooled, wrapped in steel and stored. The least dangerous solid wastes are buried at Drigg, a few miles from Sellafield, while the 'low-level' liquids are filtered to remove radioactive compounds before they make their way along a pipe into the Irish Sea.

What has added heat to the nuclear debate is the construction of a new reprocessing plant known as THORP. Shirley pointed out some grey and pink shapes in the middle distance, large wide aggregations of building blocks where reprocessing took place. THORP, not quite visible on their far side, was still idle, its work delayed by official inquiries. There were concerns about the radiation that it would give off and about the amount of waste that would be imported into West Cumbria to take advantage of the new technology. The counter-argument was that THORP was a state-of-the-art reprocessor and not to use it would threaten the survival of the whole Sellafield plant. The local papers I had seen were anxious about the huge blow that would be caused to employment in the district if THORP was not allowed to do its job.

We reached the offices of occupational health and stood in the waiting area until Dr Wood arrived. I had become so windswept that at first glance he mistook me for one of the site workers, walked on and introduced himself to Shirley. We settled into his office.

What I initially took to be apprehension in Robin Wood turned out to be laryngitis. Nevertheless he gave the impression that he did not relish the high profile that went with his work. He felt concerned for a workforce who had been made over-anxious. He disliked the way anti-nuclear arguments seemed designed to frighten people – environmentalists again. There had been times when he had found it hard to reassure them with balanced information: whipped-up fears against his own inconclusive facts; it was not a fair fight.

Robin Wood had worked for seven years to create a model occupational health service in what he believed to be the most health-conscious of industries. He had developed a treatment centre for minor injuries that resembled a modern casualty department. He had shut down an old-fashioned operating theatre originally intended to be used in urgent cases by surgeons rushed there from Cumbria hospitals. It had once been thought that accident victims who might be contaminated with radioactivity should be treated on site rather than transferred to a general hospital where they might emit radiation and endanger others; now hospitals in the area had safety procedures that allowed them to handle such cases. It had been Dr Wood too who had ended annual medical examinations, once carried out routinely on everyone, even healthy men in their twenties. It was a wasteful, indiscriminate system that has now been replaced by less frequent but more thorough checks on general health and fitness. He had explained the risks of radiation and emphasized the importance of limited exposure to it until Sellafield employees had become what he called 'the best educated workforce in the world'. Yet his practice was dominated by an illness he never had to diagnose: leukaemia.

In 1990, after Gardner had suggested that the amount of radiation received by men at Sellafield was related to the risk of leukaemia in their children, Robin Wood's clinic had seen a steady stream of worried workers.

'In the Gardner Report there was a one-liner about genetic mutation caused by radiation acting on the fathers' sperm but it was the part that everyone heard about. People working here asked me whether the same sort of genetic damage could have caused other conditions in their families – other cancers, eczema, asthma, miscarriage. They were used to worrying about themselves but the problem wasn't their own risk any more; they were worrying about the unconceived child. Men came to me in a distressed state. I had a letter from Canada from someone who hadn't worked here for years. There's less concern now but occasionally people thinking of starting a family still ask about it.'

Later I checked the 'one-liner' which turned out to be rather more, in fact the crux of Gardner's report, in his opinion the likeliest explanation for his main finding. But it may still have been true that the alarm that followed was unjustified because researchers in Ontario who tried to reproduce Gardner's results among Canadian nuclear workers could not do so. And in the most recent Sellafield study, the one that up-dated and added to the original Black Report, all the new cases had been conceived *before* their families had moved to Seascale. Damaged sperm could not have been the cause.

Instead of doing what he had wanted to do and spending his time planning the future of his blossoming service, Robin has found himself on television discussing childhood cancer with Professor Gardner or defending the Sellafield plant at public meetings.

'People say, "Here is an excess of a condition known to be caused by radiation, situated next to a nuclear power station, and you're saying the two aren't connected?" And I have to say, "There's no evidence." They find it hard to believe. I think it would be easier if I thought they were right. Then I could say, "There *is* a problem. And this is what we're doing about it."'

No evidence? With high rates of leukaemia found not only around Sellafield but near other nuclear sites such as Dounreay and Aldermaston? Yet there is an argument – a powerful scientific one – in defence of the nuclear industry and it runs like this: no one doubts that there is a cluster of childhood leukaemia in Seascale but the cause is unknown. The amount of radiation emitted from Sellafield is too small to account for it; the number of cases at each site around the country bears no relation to the size of radioactive discharges; no such clusters are found in other countries; and the genetic mutation theory has not been supported by subsequent research.

There are numerous natural sources of radiation including food, water and air. The average dose received each year by people living in the UK is 2.4 units, about half of it inhaled as radioactive gases present in small amounts in the atmosphere. Nuclear power stations add minute quantities to this total across the whole country but even in Seascale the contribution from this source is minor: 0.4 units at the most, only a sixth of all environmental radiation. This is roughly the same amount that would be received by someone who lived permanently at the top of one of the mountains in the Lake District where cosmic radiation is at least twice what it is at sea level. It is also equivalent to the radiation reaching someone spending a month's holiday in Cornwall where the environmental dose is by far the highest in Britain. So the residents of Seascale receive only a fraction of their annual radiation intake from Sellafield. How could radioactive emissions into the environment be the cause of the leukaemia cluster?

Then there is the absence of a proportionate relationship between the amount of radiation in a place and the number of cases of leukaemia, the lack of a dose–response effect, to use the scientific jargon. When trying to relate a medical finding to a possible cause, researchers look for something more than a simple link, which could be coincidental. For example, the association of lung cancer and smoking is strengthened by the fact that the more you smoke, the higher the risk of cancer. The same applies to liver cirrhosis and alcohol. But it is not true that the number of cases of leukaemia around Britain's numerous nuclear installations is related to the amount of radiation they each release. At Sellafield alone there has been no decline in leukaemia to go with the reduction in emission since the 1970s. And to confound the research, an excess of leukaemia has also been reported in some places where nuclear power stations were planned but not built, raising the possibility that something else about the sites where they are usually placed may hold the answer.

All this has been enough for Robin Wood. 'No reputable scientist believes environmental radiation is the cause,' he told me. 'There is no dose–response effect which there would be if emissions were to blame. After all we are talking about something measurable – physical energy, not magic moonbeams. If there was a relationship with the radiation coming from here, you'd be able to show it.' Dr Wood had no doubt about his own safety or that of his family and I was about to ask if that meant he would be prepared to live in Seascale when he volunteered that he did. 'There's so much concern about leukaemia,' he said with a hint of irony, 'but the best thing I could do for the health of the workforce would be to stop them smoking.'

Robin gave me a printed sheet listing what his medical duties were and we went outside to his car and headed for the building where injuries that could be radioactive were examined. I glanced at the list. It included advising on the medical suitability of prospective employees. 'They have to be able to run if there's a problem of criticality,' he said, a reference to the critical mass of uranium that is the trigger for a nuclear detonation. I studied his expression for signs that he was joking. 'Not that there would be an explosion here but there would be an enormous pulse of energy in the form of gamma radiation.'

The list also mentioned a twenty-four hour service for employees who became contaminated. The clinic was on the border between high and low radioactivity areas, a crossing point from the part of Sellafield where radioactive materials were handled into the safer world of lower radiation. No one was allowed to leave the 'active' area without being checked for contamination and this was equally true of those who had been hurt in accidents. The border itself ran through the clinic, separating the room where people were initially taken after an incident from another where treatment took place, the dividing line between them being a low-lying desk of the sort you find in a left luggage office.

Two sorts of incident brought the workforce to the radioactive side of the clinic. Usually someone would be routinely checking their hands for contamination at the end of the day's shift when they would unexpectedly find that radiation could be detected. Or else the victim of a not-so-serious industrial accident would be brought or sent so that their wound could be examined for 'activity'. The clinic was in action many times every week.

When we arrived there was a skinny man of about twenty with a sulky sidelong glance waiting to be seen by the clinic nurse. There was a graze on his hand. From the antechamber on the radioactive side he was directed into a man-size lead cubicle designed to cut out background radiation; a kind of Geiger counter was run across the injured patch of skin. The worst type of radioactivity to have in a wound is alpha radiation, although in other circumstances it is the least troublesome as it cannot penetrate skin and enter the body. Once inside an open cut, however, alpha-emitting material can lodge itself in the body, the liver or the bones particularly, where the qualities that normally keep its rays out of living tissue are equally effective in keeping them in. People who turn up positive on the Geiger counter must have their wounds cleaned or their skin scrubbed. One of the clinic rooms contains two showers for this purpose as well as a basin with a concave neck rest for those whose hair has to be thoroughly de-contaminated. Sometimes the outer layer of dead skin on the hands has to be removed and to ensure that none is missed the skin is first stained with potassium permanganate – the purple solution in a child's chemistry set – before a corrosive liquid is applied, removing the stain and the radioactive epidermis. All the discarded materials from these operations, the paper towels and the water used in rinsing, is low-level waste and, like the leftovers from reprocessing, it too is buried at Drigg or piped into the sea.

There were no clicks of radiation from the man's wound: he was cleared to pass through to the treatment room. I was ready to leave, having seen and heard what I was there for. Robin drove me back to where we had started and it seemed the right time to bring up something more personal. How had he come to be a doctor in the nuclear business, I asked.

'I was a GP, then I was in another industry in occupational health. But I had always been interested in nuclear power. When I was a child I was fascinated by the idea of splitting the atom. Where I used to work, people were taking real risks and no one said anything. Now I'm in one of the safest industries there is and there's all this anxiety. But I'm happy to show people what I do. I don't really mind what you write, even if it's critical.'

But there was nothing to criticize in the way all worries were dismissed in Sellafield because, as far as they go, the denials are indisputable. The cases of leukaemia and lymphoma at Seascale could not have been caused by the level of radiation in the local environment as it is currently understood, so the radioactivity known to be seeping out of Sellafield could not have been responsible. And the link with the dose of radiation received by fathers is limited to a single uncorroborated study while later evidence goes the other way. Nothing to criticize but something to be surprised about: the certainty in the individuals I had met but apparently also in the surrounding towns that there is no risk from the nuclear plant despite an outbreak of illness that is unexplained. It was hard for me to feel so reassured while the real culprit was unknown and at large.

But that did not seem to me to be the end of the medical story at Sellafield because the extent of the public furore needs its own explanation. Even if nuclear power stations did cause leukaemia, the threat to the general population would be tiny in comparison to many other causes of illness. Five thousand people are killed on the roads every year in Britain but protesters do not chain themselves to the fences of car factories and academic research into road safety does not make headline news. Something about the nuclear threat to health must touch a raw nerve to produce such an outcry.

It can not be simply that, while we feel in control of how we drive, we are at the mercy of radiation, because our control does not extend to how other people drive. The fears must lie in the nature of the threat itself. It is invisible and insidious, characteristics it has in common with Aids or even BSE, illnesses that have provoked similar public dread. What terrifies us about radiation is not just what it can cause but its clandestine approach, the way it sneaks into us unseen and lies in wait, ready for the unpredictable moment in the future when it will strike us down. In this it has much in common not only with the most alarming of modern diseases but with the plagues and epidemics that used to devastate the population before their microscopic cause was found. It is an old fear in a new guise.

I was soon back on Stoneside Hill and driving east with a mountainous horizon ahead of me in the early evening sky. I had seen the meticulous attention to safety at Sellafield but I had still been troubled by what we had discussed. The detailed descriptions of safety precautions and the elaborate methods of waste disposal had had a contrary, illogical, effect. Like the out-of-the-way location, it all left me more rather than less uneasy and I was glad to be leaving. On these twisted roads I wanted to put some miles behind me before it was dark. I preferred to see anything that might be dangerous.

SIX

Belfast

THE BEST travel writing comes out of trains: the human drama and sloth squeezed in the same carriage, and the endless reel of the passing world outside, force the passive writer into observation. Planes are poor rivals because they have nothing to show except a succession of towns in miniature. But the flight into Belfast is different. Suddenly the city's western ghettos appear through dirty clouds: cramped, featureless and stuck where Louis MacNiece jammed his birthplace, 'between the mountain and the gantries'.

At the road block on the city approach route from the airport, the car I was in slowed momentarily until armed police waved us through in the direction of the town. I had never visited Belfast before but I knew the names of its districts as they appeared on road signs: Andersontown, Shankill, Turf Lodge, Ballymurphy. Up above the motorway that slices through the city I saw the Divis flats, a solitary tower block on the evening skyline, mounted with an army look-out.

Then, within minutes, we were in a suburb the colour of autumn, stopping among gardens and university halls and stepping into a cool night. The atmosphere in the bar was noisy and thick with the smell of beer as we entered and ordered. This was where the staff of Queen's University came to mix with each other but it could have been an academics' watering hole anywhere in Britain, except that it was louder.

'Do you want to know the real story about Northern Ireland?', Peter Curran asked me when the drinks arrived. I did. 'Resilience. That's all there is to know.'

I met no shortage of people over the next two days who would tell me the same thing, that Belfast, despite its political turmoil, was like every other town of its size, full of shoppers and pubs, with too much litter and not enough clean air. They would even insist that, for all the deaths of the last twenty or so years, it outstripped other cities with its roaring enjoyment of life. Where it wasn't genteel – and some of its suburbs looked as prim as a finishing school – it was gloriously drunk. It bustled and buzzed and argued and, if you were lucky enough to know it, really know it, you could never leave because no other city would do. Its vitality was unique and even had its own name: people stayed here for the *crack* of the place.

The crack is resilience by another name and you could also hear it in the local brogue. Many people find the Ulster accent harsh, like an expression of resentment over the continual rain, as if the weather was a personal affront. But its tone is tougher than that; it is not an accent that goes with indecision or doubt but one of survival.

Resilience is also the most obvious message of research into the psychological impact of the civil war. Cars have exploded in busy streets, civilians have been shot in error, the army patrols the estates, the public have been interned and terrorized. But there has been no flooding of hospitals and GP surgeries with mental disorders. There has been no mass demand for tranquillizers and no dramatic upsurge in suicide.

In the early days of the conflict, there were reports of rising rates of parasuicide (non-fatal self-harm) but they are now discounted. In the 1960s and 1970s parasuicide hit the UK as an epidemic, becoming the second commonest cause of admission to medical beds (second to heart disease) and if there really was an increase in Northern Ireland, it was probably no more than was happening nationwide. Research suggests that Ulster people who take overdoses, the method used by 90 per cent of parasuicides, do so in response to the same traumas as anywhere in the country – broken relationships, family arguments and lost jobs – and not to the stress of the conflict. The parasuicides themselves do not blame the troubles.

Suicide rates even fell as the violence began, and fell dramatically. This would not have been surprising to Emile Durkheim, a French sociologist, who at the turn of the century revealed that suicide rates around 1850 had diminished in those European countries where there had been political upheaval. He argued that conflict made societies more cohesive by confronting them with a common enemy, and that the strong social ties that resulted were protective to vulnerable individuals who might otherwise kill themselves. During this century the suicide rate in Britain did what Durkheim would have predicted, and fell during both World Wars. In fact it dropped steadily year by year but dipped abruptly in the war years. In 1969 Northern Ireland began its latest resurgence of internal war and in 1970 the suicide rate in the province fell by half.

Durkheim would have said that each side of the conflict was now bound together by its opposition to the other. But there was another possible explanation which a better-known guru might have supported: Sigmund Freud would have pointed to the rising murder rate which coincided with the drop in suicide. He believed that depression was the result of aggressive feelings directed inward and by his theory a falling suicide rate was a product of the social violence that made it possible to express hostility outwardly.

A third way of accounting for the decline is to fall back on a common style of scientific question: *Compared to what* was the suicide rate low in Northern Ireland in the early 1970s? Answer: compared to the rate in the late 1960s. But this rate was unusually high, so the subsequent figures represented a steeper reduction than would be seen if a longer view of the fluctuations was taken. But why was the rate in the late 1960s so inflated? Could it have been because of social tension for which the violence proved cathartic? Whatever the truth was, it wasn't the truth for long, as any difference between Ulster and the rest of the UK soon disappeared. By the mid-1970s, suicide in the Six Counties was rising slowly, as it was throughout the country.

But gross statistics camouflage details, and to look at the health of the entire province risks missing any variation within it. Northern Ireland as a whole may not have collapsed into a flurry of self-poisoning or a blur of tranquillizers but there are many parts of the country which have barely been touched by the conflict. How can anyone be sure that there are not also pockets of distress and illness where the violence most often strikes? If so, the estates of West Belfast would be affected worst of all.

Peter Curran is a psychiatrist whose hospital, the Mater Infirmorum, stands at the east end of Crumlin Road, an old Catholic infirmary a hundred metres from the heart of Shankill, the largest of the Protestant districts in the west sector of the city. Much of the research into the mental ill health of the Northern Ireland conflict is his work, some of it carried out together with Gerry Loughrey, with whom he was now collaborating on a project to buy more Guinness than I could drink.

Peter gave me the impression that self-doubt did not usually slow him down. He had guessed who I was from all the passengers emerging from my plane. He never paused for long at the army road blocks. It was a trait that must have made him attractive to lawyers in another area of his work, which was litigation and the judgement of disability.

Compensation is a thriving industry in Ireland. 'We are a highly litigious folk,' Peter Curran told me. 'If there's a paving stone out of place in Belfast, it's amazing how many people will fall over it. If a bomb goes off in the city, there can be five hundred claims for psychological injury.'

If resilience is one of the themes of Belfast's psychology, the toughness of a whole society that prevents it from disintegrating, then another is the awful vulnerability of individuals caught up in the fight. Dr Curran had seen many of them, people who had survived a brush with death but whose lives were in ruins.

'I wrote a report on a man the other day. He answered a knock at the door but there was no one there so he stepped out on to the pavement to look around. About twenty yards away he saw someone kneeling, pointing a gun at him. He tried to run away along the street but he was hit in the leg and fell. He lay there unable to move, listening to the gunman's footsteps getting nearer and waiting to be shot again. Then for some reason – maybe he looked as if he was already dead – the gunman turned and ran.'

For the men to whom these things happen, the initial terrifying trauma is only the beginning. 'After that he was too afraid to return home. He moved away for his own protection and in effect lost his wife, his family and his job. And he's an example of a survivor.

'Something similar happened to an RUC man I examined. He told me he had learned to live with the constant risk that anything in a street could explode as he was walking past it. For years he had looked under cars and stayed clear of litter bins, so that it had become routine. He thought he knew all the places where bombs might be hidden. But one day he was patrolling a street in formation and he had to stop. There was nothing suspicious that he could see but a small amount of Semtex had been attached to a lamppost next to where he was standing and it blew him across the road. The point is that he recovered from his injuries but his confidence has completely gone and he'll never work again.'

The next morning, after breakfast with a troupe of noisy student actors, I left the University Staff Club and took a walk in the direction of Donegal Square, in the centre of the town. I wanted to witness firsthand the atmosphere and the structure of the place, to sample it for clues to the essence of resilience, to find out more about how a society stayed sane when parts of it were tearing each other to pieces.

The shoppers in the city centre could have been excused if they were feeling edgy. It was a nervous time in Northern Ireland, though admittedly one of many. A few days before, civilians in different parts of the province had been coerced into driving cars loaded with explosives into army checkpoints and the horror of these incidents had been big news, not only because of what took place but because of what they were thought to signify. Could it mean an end to a longstanding IRA policy of attacking only 'legitimate' targets and so begin a new period of danger for people not otherwise involved in the conflict? At the same time, there had been a number of what the press calls – in the playground slang that is used to take the sting out of such events – 'tit-for-tat' killings in West Belfast and other districts in which the victims of the Loyalist gangs had been selected at random. It was no longer possible for large sections of the population to believe this was somebody else's battle.

The early 1970s had been the era of car bombs in public places. The centre of major towns had suffered badly, being both physically destroyed and commercially undermined as the threat of explosions deterred businesses and customers alike. But since around 1975, when the Provisional IRA switched its sights more exclusively to the army and police, the centre of Belfast had been regenerated. But could it survive if there was to be a further change of target?

It seemed that morning like a city with somewhere to go, a self-confident city. The main entrance to the shopping precinct was guarded by a security fence and two genial police officers with the air of janitors. Once inside people jostled and browsed their way round new stores and arcades, pausing occasionally for the ritual search of pockets and handbags by security men. It did not look like a city afraid of violence. When workmen threw a cement block into a skip on Donegal Street, I was the only person who jumped. Its atmosphere was of urban normality.

But passing along Bedford Street on the way out of the centre I became aware that something was going on ahead of me. Pedestrians were crossing to the opposite pavement and cars were being stopped and questioned. There were soldiers with automatic weapons in the road and in doorways, checking vehicles and taking up position down side streets. This too was normal in Belfast and a hint of what I was to see later that day.

Peter Curran had arranged for me to meet two psychiatrists, Graeme McDonald and Philip McGarry. Graeme was in charge of community services for West Belfast and Philip was soon to join him in the task. Medicine in Ulster's capital is dominated, like many other aspects of life, by Ulster people. Few outsiders seek employment here and indigenous locals take advantage of the resulting ease of promotion. Little of the interchange of doctors and others that takes place elsewhere in the country occurs in Northern Ireland but the positive consequence is that those who reach senior positions often know the country and the population well.

And vice versa. Graeme's tiny car was, he told me, a familiar sight around his patch of the city. Even the Provisional IRA, he believed, had his registration number on a computer file it kept to identify cars entering the district. To me it was an amazing idea that paramilitary records might include the neighbourhood's psychiatrist but, as it was in no one's interest to deter health personnel from doing their work, it made perfect sense. And it was a relief to know it as we hurtled round West Belfast's ramshackle estates, reversed down cul-de-sacs and stopped from time to time for the others to point something out to me. A suspicious sight we must have made, three men in a car, looking and pointing. And suspicious we certainly were to judge from the wary looks we received, though in Graeme's opinion the worst thing that could happen to us was that we could be mistaken for yet another television crew. Still, I hoped the IRA look-outs had managed a good view of our number-plate.

Although West Belfast is mainly Catholic its northern edge is the firmly Protestant district of Shankill and there are islands of Protestant housing scattered elsewhere within it. This close proximity combined with the ingrained hostility between the two religions has been the source of much of the trouble and in many places territorial barriers have been erected by the security forces: tall corrugated fences that loom like prison walls across streets and beside gardens. On one side of these 'peace lines' the pavement kerb has been painted red, white and blue, on the other the green, white and orange of the Irish tricolour.

Most of the pavements were in Republican colours as we sped from Falls in the north to Andersontown in the south and back again. It was a macabre tour. Some of the places we passed, ordinary suburban streets with local stores and bus queues, had been the setting for notorious killings. We halted at the frequently photographed mural of figures in paramilitary uniform and came across an occasional memorial at the end of a terrace, painted with the names and ranks of dead members of the IRA. At the end of one street there was a police station, impossible to see clearly through its dense barrier of protective mesh.

If the violence did have a geographically restricted effect on the mental health of people living close to it, this was where it would be manifest. In fact one survey of the prescribing of tranquillizers by West Belfast GPs found substantial increases after the initial riots in 1969. But whether this tightly localized upturn was maintained once sporadic violence had become the norm is not known. In any case some of the psychological trauma may make its appearance only after a lengthy period of apparent coping, which makes it hard for researchers to detect. Delayed reactions of this sort, known as post-traumatic stress disorder, have been much publicized in American veterans of Vietnam, some of whom suffered anxiety, nightmares and flashbacks long after returning home. Similar disturbances have been found by Peter Curran's collaborator, Gerry Loughrey, in people exposed to the war in Belfast, and many of the victims, their distress often unrecognized, must live in the area I was now viewing. But the origins of mental disorder cannot be separated from the social conditions in which it arises. Unemployment, often linked to depression, is higher in Ulster than in most parts of the United Kingdom. And the housing, another contributor to misery and a marker for the poverty that both causes and amplifies despair, is bleak.

I lost track of where we were several times, so similar were the rows of houses and the tortuous streets around the estates. Only the bare hill to the north-west, by acting as a marker, revealed which direction we were facing, and I could make out near its summit the beginnings of a political slogan, the word 'Free' and a trace of another letter, daubed or laid out in stone; it was impossible from that distance to tell which.

There are those, I was aware, who blame the social and political neglect still evident in West Belfast for the civil war itself, not simply for compounding its psychiatric consequences. Its beginnings, they say, were a civil rights movement demanding political and economic freedom and its solution could still lie in improving the lot of the disfranchised minority, thus draining the resentment which acts as fertile ground for paramilitary sympathy.

But analysis based on class and suffrage are mistaken, however tempting they sometimes seem to those who find inequality a more acceptable basis for social unrest. The only distinction that matters in Belfast is the religious one, from which everything else stems. A civil conflict quickly takes on the shape of its society's most fundamental division and the battle lines in Northern Ireland, though initially they may have separated two sides of a dispute over rights, were soon replaced by peace lines between Catholics and Protestants. In fact there has been an attempt to modernize the housing of West Belfast and relieve some of the environmental hardship, but it has had no noticeable impact on the violence.

Yet there are aspects of social disadvantage, poor housing being one, that transcend the sectarian divide and make the Protestant area of Shankill almost indistinguishable from Ballymurphy, Falls and the others. Only the colour of the pavements and the bias of the graffiti are different. Peter Curran even went so far as to attribute – tentatively – the absence of any epidemic of mental illness to the common features of the two religious cultures. Each was under threat, albeit from the other, and the shared sense of being under siege provided the two communities with a protective cohesion. This was more than saying, as Durkheim would, that the two sides were rendered more supportive to their own members because of each other's opposition; it was suggesting that there was an unexpressed mutual support between Protestants and Catholics arising from their identical predicament.

The similarities between the two religions were not hard to find. From the next street we heard the roll of a drum and a few snatches of flute, in Ulster the sound of religious bigotry. When we reached the source of the music, the band was preparing to march and a group of RUC officers in bullet-proof jackets were holding up traffic to let it pass. We were in Shankill so the musicians were Protestant but Philip said that a similar event in Catholic West Belfast would look the same except that there would be no police. Or else the duty of supervision might be performed by the Provisionals.

The authority asssumed by the IRA in West Belfast is extensive, covering business, transport and policing, and even including those areas of crime on which psychiatrists are often called in for advice, such as sexual offences and adolescent recidivism. The Provisionals are firmly embedded in the part of the city from where they operate. Only on their say-so can taxi-drivers or builders work in the area and no one dares to rob the stores they smile on.

It is a conservative authority that they exercise, so much so that teenagers rebel against it, usually to their cost. Among Belfast's youth joy-riding is a common sport and it is said that the IRA takes a tough line with those who do it too often. Whereas in other cities in the UK recalcitrant car thieves might find themselves in the hands of child psychologists, here they may have to face the local paramilitaries. Sex offenders too, those who expose themselves or commit assaults, who might in other places be assessed by forensic psychiatrists, are reputedly looked on with special distaste.

The injuries it is said that the Provisionals inflict on those who step out of line have had one benefit. Although the infamous knee-capping is apparently quite rare, gunshot wounds to the limbs as well as assorted broken bones are not, and the medical services of Belfast have developed a pioneering expertise in their treatment. The years of civil war have left the city's hospitals richly skilled in dealing with the trauma caused by bomb blasts and bullets of both high and low velocity. Emergency services, neurosurgery, orthopaedics and vascular surgery have all responded to the war by developing new and rapid techniques of treating casualties and have become recognized worldwide as leaders in their fields. It is another side to Ulster's resilience.

Much of this medical success has been achieved at the Royal Victoria Hospital where our motorized excursion now ended and a pedestrian tour began. I wanted to see the estates close up rather than at high speed, and a walk through Falls and Shankill was agreed. Only half-way through did Philip tell me he had never before ventured into this part of the city on foot.

The lanes seemed narrower and the rows of houses tinier and more ancient than they had earlier and most streets were empty except where children were playing or, in one place, throwing stones at each other. In the first years of the civil war there was some evidence that the children of Belfast were suffering from emotional disorders as a result of the conflict but this has not been confirmed by a plethora of more recent research. Like adults they have in general seemed more stolid than might have been predicted, although that is not necessarily a source of comfort. After all, the most convincing way of accounting for how impervious they seem to be to the horrors in their neighbourhood is to say that they have grown accustomed to them – habituated, in the language of psychology. This means that they are unmoved by violence of a certain severity and that to upset them requires something more shocking, such as direct involvement. Even though this muted reaction is primarily protective, it seems also to be inherently undesirable.

Experimenters have also found that children, while not overtly harmed by the conflict, are selectively conscious of it. Asked to write about violence, children living in Belfast are generally more able than children from a peaceful part of the province to give examples of all types, from bombs to killing birds. The rural children see violence largely as something that happens in other places, and specifically in

Belfast. Within West Belfast Catholic children are more likely than their Protestant neighbours to refer to shootings and riots, yet only a small minority of all children mention violence between religions. And when given a more oblique task, to write about where they live, only half of them mention violence at all.

We were still in the Catholic estates when Graeme chose to make an unwelcome reference to it himself. This was the sort of place, he said, where people were shot at random. In the recent killings by Loyalists the victims had simply been encountered in a Catholic area and so assumed to be suitable targets. If his family knew he was walking here, said Graeme, they would be horrified. We quickened our pace, reached an electronically-controlled gate and headed finally into Shankill. Graeme told us, 'This is where I grew up,' and at the same moment a child appeared from a doorway and prodded my leg with a plastic fork.

The slogans on the miniature terraced houses had switched allegiance. Here they daubed '1690', the date of the Battle of the Boyne, where the Protestant William of Orange defeated the Catholic James II. William, I had already found, had invaded Britain when James and his wife, after visiting Bath, had conceived a Catholic heir to the throne. It was odd to think that this date, trumpeted wherever Protestant bigotry exists, would have meant nothing without the procreative power of spa water. Another frequent slogan was 'Ulster says no'. Philip remarked, 'Ulster always says no, whatever the question.'

Minutes later, passing an elaborate wall painting of Loyalist para-military groups, we stepped out on to Crumlin Road and along to the Mater Infirmorum, the hospital where we were to be picked up. Ironically this old Catholic infirmary serves the adjacent Protestant neighbourhood and is apparently highly popular with it, a reminder that the cheek-by-jowl existence of Catholics and Protestants has produced individual friendships across the religious boundary as well as collective animosity.

That evening I was taken by friends out to a public bar in East Belfast, though there was nothing public about the place. It was a Protestant drinking-den with no external clue to what went on inside other than a few words written on the lintel. As we entered, a man lounging near the doorway stood up and politely blocked our path. One of the people I was with, however, had been here before and after a nod of recognition we were in.

The room filled up rapidly with customers who knew each other. Drinks and more drinks were drunk, voices were raised and eventually the singing started. I had been in Belfast not much more than twenty-four hours and was due to leave the following morning but it felt much longer. I had seen some of the city's strengths and some of its desperate weaknesses. I had walked from one hospital that had been spurred by the civil war into breaking new medical ground to another that proved the compatibility of two communities that refused to be reconciled.

That these were both components of Ulster's resilience I had no doubt, as was the way the people were strengthened by facing adversity together and the fact that even young children could simply grow used to violence in their vicinity. But there was another angle to the resilience story and that was how much everyone wanted it to be true, how everyone I met believed it and seemed ready to go on believing it regardless of what might happen. One of Ulster's strengths, it seemed to me, was how determined it was to look strong and the day it dropped its imperturbable posture, the day it stopped caring how it impressed the outside world with its refusal to be ruffled, was the day it would be in serious trouble.

For the crack of the place to survive it needed a hefty amount of denial, the capacity to push anything unacceptable to the back of its mind, to believe not just in its survival but in its success and to ignore all contradictory evidence. Denial was at the heart of Belfast's toughness. For some people it was an effortless process aided by living away from any genuine danger, while for others it could be sustained only by some determined turning of a blind eye to reality. Sitting in the middle of a sectarian sing-song I thought of the previous night spent in the packed University bar. 'There are folk out there trying to blow us up,' Peter Curran had shouted, 'and we're in here having a drink. Now that's denial.'

SEVEN

The Outer Hebrides

'PEOPLE here don't like being written about,' I was warned on Harris. 'Books about the Hebrides don't go down well.' I asked why not. 'Because they always come up with the same easy caricature. We drink too much, we're dominated by the Church and we're dirty.' Once in a while the islanders take their revenge. There is one Hebridean travelogue full of meetings with islanders no one knows, who say things no one believes.

But at least its author got there. Many creative artists, even those whose names are famously linked to the islands, never crossed to the far side of the Minch, the sea being too rough for the small boats that were once the only means of travel. Rough seas meant that Felix Mendelssohn wrote his 'Hebrides' overture without setting foot in the outer isles. To Samuel Johnson the islands seemed so inaccessible that he compared them to Borneo and halted his island-hopping on Skye. There he met Flora Macdonald, who had taken Bonnie Prince Charlie back across the Minch from North Uist and thus inspired the Hebridean Boat Song, which you can still sing along to on any Western Isles ferry; it is a favoured piece of muzak.

Someone who did go all the way was Halliday Sutherland, a doctor who in 1939 published his *Hebridean Journey*, an account of how he visited most of the inhabited islands in the five hundred-strong archipelago, collecting tales of witches and herring, and dining at the tables of island gentry. On Harris they disapprove of him without really meaning it. Halliday was fond of a good story, I heard, and he didn't lose sleep over whether or not it was true.

Dr Sutherland reached Tarbert, Harris's only town, at two in the morning and 'in darkness with a drizzle of rain', having taken a boat from Loch Maddy, a sea loch at the top corner of North Uist. When I landed in Tarbert fifty years later it was still raining. I had spent the previous night on the north-west coast of Skye, in Uig, which is Gaelic for bay. But when I had looked out of my hotel window that morning, the bay had vanished. A dense mist had swallowed it and looked set to linger for days, though within an hour it had cleared to make way for a fine, penetrating rain carried by the first puffs of what was soon to be a hurricane.

When the Bonnie Prince escaped across the Minch to Benbecula after the massacre at Culloden, he was so seasick that he said afterwards he would rather have faced the Duke of Cumberland's cannon. But the boat that ferried me to Tarbert was stable enough to collide with a tidal wave without spilling breakfast. In any case neither the wind nor the wet were severe during the crossing and, two hours later, as we glided between the tiny islands of East Loch Tarbert, I had through the rain a clear view of Scalpay, the largest of them and my immediate destination.

I wanted to go there because I had given in to an impulse that must seize many a Hebridean traveller, to go one island further. All the way through the western highlands to the Kyle of Lochalsh, then on to Skye and across to its northern peninsula, I had felt a growing sense of remoteness and the liberation that goes with it. Skye had lain across the narrow Kyle at first, then it was behind me and from it I had seen Harris at the horizon. Now in Tarbert I was keen to reach another island. If I could drive the five miles east along the single track road to Carnach, I would be in time for the only ferry to Scalpay for several hours.

Remoteness was what had brought me to the Outer Hebrides, to witness it in person, to observe its effect on medicine and medical folk and to ask the latter what possessed them to live there. Was life on Harris all whisky and Genesis? A local GP whose practice spread over twenty miles from its centre in Tarbert had said yes to a meeting later in the day and would have the answer.

No one was around when I reached the ferry pier that pointed over the Sound of Scalpay to the island itself but a line of empty vehicles in a short lay-by showed where to park. There was one space left and I backed into it and then, to a grunt from the car, into the running stream behind it. It was a half-space, it was a concealed drop, it was too short for a car, but it was a pretty stream.

The vehicle was now partly up-ended, resting its chassis on the edge of the bank with its back wheels tipping towards the water a metre below. I examined the tiny cottages which constitute Carnach, trying to guess which of them was the best bet for a breakdown truck. But just then luck arrived in the form of a jeep whose driver glanced at where the back of my car was aiming.

'It looks as if you've reversed too far,' he offered.

'It looks as if I have.'

The accent was English but the desiccated tone was pure island. He drove on, backed up, fixed a rope between us, pulled me out, and then spoke again. I had been caught looking at the pile of ropes and chains he was carrying and I suppose he felt he should explain. It was all down to the weather forecast. There had been a warning of strong gales and the man with the chains was going to Scalpay to tie everything down. It was likely to be 'a real hooler,' he said, enjoying – as all expatriates do – the use of a local word. The warning spoke of force twelve, hurricane strength, but everyone I met for the rest of the day predicted force eleven. The forecast, they shrugged, was known to exaggerate.

Whatever the number, it was a hurricane by name. This was Isadora, fresh from the Caribbean and not yet blown out. The Hebrides are used to strong winds. Their fishermen habitually go out in them, even when they reach force eight or nine. Today the trawlers were being tied down. If it was medicine in a hostile lanscape I was after, I had timed my visit well.

Scalpay is still what the whole Outer Hebrides used to be. As a society it is close rather than closed, though the two are sometimes hard to tell apart, and strong on God and fish. Herring saved the economy of the Hebrides after the infamous clearances, which were anyway made less severe in some of the Western Isles by the benevolence of James Matheson. With the money he made from trading opium in the Far East, Matheson bought Lewis, then fed and employed its population after the potato famine of 1846.

Even after the Russian Revolution slashed their market – the new republic did not want to buy herring – the islands' fishermen used to follow the shoals round the mainland coast to Leith and Lowestoft and the women, skilled in the art of gutting, would go with them. It was a tough existence and many men suffered injuries; ulcers, that plague of city executives, were frequent, allegedly from going all day without food. Young Hebrideans who would once have followed the customary path to the harbours no longer do so, preferring a less strenuous career, and who can blame them? As a result there are now almost as many fish farms as trawlers in the islands.

People say the cohesion of communities like Scalpay is primarily a legacy of fishing, that outsiders are wrong to portray it as a product of the pulpit. As a result neighbours are first to spot when someone is ill and quick to alert the doctor, acting as an early warning system which urban practitioners would certainly envy. Yet the Church plays its part as well and a family in social or marital crisis is as likely to receive a house call from a kirk elder as from a doctor.

In most parts of the highlands and isles it is the Free Presbyterian Church which dominates religious life. Although a relatively new movement, it is an old-time religion. It began in 1843 as a revolt against the established Church, whose leaders refused to defend the crofters and villagers against the landowners when the latter wanted to clear them out of their homesteads and replace them with sheep. After further in-fighting and schism, the present Free Church emerged with an abundant supply of fire and brimstone. To the outside world its image is of bowler-hatted puritans torturing any red-blooded parishioner with a mediaeval religiosity. As I had heard, it is a reputation resented by islanders.

For every element of truth in the image there is another of distortion. Researchers who studied depression in Hebridean women a decade ago found there was less of it than in inner London and one reason was that church membership seemed to be protective. More surprising was that people I spoke to regarded the Church as tolerant in moral matters such as illegitimacy and even too tolerant of alcoholism. Despite their reputation, island communities seem to have a tradition of supporting rather than hounding that familiar target, the unmarried mother, and the 'Wee Free' save their outrage for less critical matters, such as the sanctity of the sabbath.

Even before Free Presbyterianism, the Church was not slow to speak its mind. When Bonnie Prince Charlie sheltered on Scalpay, the Minister for Harris, Aulay Macaulay, great-grandfather of the nineteenth-century historian, tried to capture him and, having failed, ranted against him until no one for miles would take him in. The prince's subsequent flight in the reluctant company of Flora Macdonald became a miserable procession of disease and infestation, relieved only by the occasional prolonged swig from a brandy bottle. He went down with dysentery, was plundered by lice and sucked dry by midges. It was his last experience of Scotland.

It didn't take long to drive as far as the road would go on Scalpay. I thought of walking round to the lighthouse at Eilean Glas but the facing wind was already insistent enough to turn each step into a slow-motion plod. It even made the telegraph wires sing, as strong winds are supposed to.

The export of young people, particularly skilled people, to distant parts of the country has not only turned island communities like Scalpay old, but has deprived the growing proportion of elderly people of their traditional support. No longer are their families nearby for them to call on or move to. There are too few able-bodied neighbours to help and those who *are* fit find themselves in great demand. Medical care for the elderly, wherever they live, relies on families or social agencies acting *in loco familiae*. But on the Hebrides there is a shortage of those who might work as, for instance, home-helps. After all, if there were any people available to take that sort of job, they would already be doing it for nothing.

The cohesion of the islands has held out for generations against the intrusion of the way of life across the water and it can be tempting to see the remoteness as an asset, able to sew the seeds of community and so give the inhabitants a robustness of health and character. But once the cohesion begins to break down, as it seems to be doing under the strain of selective migration, it can very quickly fall apart.

The language of the school playground on Scalpay is itself a sign of changing times. Islanders have an emotional attachment to their own tongue and talk of 'having the Gaelic' as if it were a sixth sense. It was once outlawed in schools, which did not damage its popularity, then encouraged, which did. Most of the older people are fluent but on Scalpay the school children speak a precise Hebridean English.

The school looked as if it was being evacuated as I passed it and the cottages around the island's two harbours were tightly shuttered. They were taking no chances with Isadora. I rushed to rendezvous with the ferry that would take me back to Harris and got there early enough not to be among those who were left behind. For them the next scheduled ferry was a few hours away and, to judge by the way the wind was notching higher up the Beaufort scale with every blow, they were in danger of staying there till morning. The boat, little more than a floating platform, would not be strong enough to make the crossing and would be given a night off.

At its surface the sound was surprisingly flat, more like a cornfield in a gale than the sea, but as we crossed the half-mile stretch, water raced round the boat at both ends and pushed as if we were in the way of something important. Eventually we clattered into the row of tyres along the side of the Carnach jetty whose job was to take the impact on days like these. In less than a minute I was on the road for Tarbert and the rain was falling in torrents.

Half a century earlier Halliday Sutherland stood outside the only hotel in Tarbert in the 2 a.m. drizzle, hoping for a dry bed. How he made it from the harbour when not a single building was lit, not even the hotel itself, he doesn't say. When the hotelier finally opened his door, it was to let another late guest in and turn Halliday away, although he relented when he realized this middle-aged gent would have to sleep in a field.

From my hotel I had only a short dash to the surgery of the GP I had arranged to see but then a long wet wait outside what looked like a door but wasn't. In any case Dr Robertson was not there; his flight from Uist was delayed because of the storm, though not by much. There was also a rumour around the hotel that the next morning's ferry would be unable to sail, although the staff were doubtful that the wind would live up to its advance publicity.

John Robertson was soft-spoken and polite and would have been at home in one of A. J. Cronin's fictional surgeries, so exactly did he portray the Highland bedside manner. Yet medicine was his second career and he had entered it, quite literally, by accident. He had begun his working life as a fisherman out of Fraserburgh but when as a young man at sea his forearm was smashed, he left the boats, believing he could not pull his weight beside his fellow seamen. The accident, I was intrigued to hear, had taken place a few miles from where we were talking, in West Loch Tarbert, the other side of the pincer of seawater that would cut Harris in two if it were not for the isthmus where Tarbert holds it together.

Why, it was impossible not to ask, had he come back – and as a doctor – to the very place where the progress of his life had been re-routed for medical reasons? Dr Robertson saw nothing meaningful in that.

'I had just qualified. A job came up here and I applied for it.'

I was sceptical. 'But why here? Why didn't you apply for one somewhere else, like Birmingham?' It seemed an obvious question.

'I did. I got a job in Birmingham but turned it down because I didn't like the town. I went for a walk with my wife down a street called – coincidentally – Aberdeen Street and we realized this wasn't what we wanted.'

It could have been the name that put him off, I suggested. Aberdeen, like Fraserburgh, is one of the fishing ports of the north-east coast. It was part of his old life, now replaced by a new career in medicine, and therefore rejected. Yet since then his two vocations had been linked, like the two parts of Harris itself, by the town of Tarbert, where he had first lost his fishing career and then set up his medical practice. But Dr Robertson didn't think so.

The economic development of the Hebrides has altered his work and not always in ways he has welcomed. Until recently there was no road to the village of Rhenigdale on the east coast of Harris, so any house call there meant a six-mile walk along a fairly mountainous footpath. If the weather was rough or the call urgent, he would be collected by fishermen from Scalpay and transported round the headland. The challenge of the inclement terrain was something he enjoyed and he took pleasure in turning up out of the sea with his black bag. But he recognized that for many islanders the old ways of living, without the mod cons he called 'gadgets', were physically tough.

There are two sides to the breaking down of traditions. One is a less arduous life-style, the other is a disintegrating culture, and each has its equivalent in health care. With the development of the islands has come easier access to treatment because of new roads, an improved hospital in Stornoway and an air-ambulance service to carry those with serious injuries or less common diseases to larger medical centres in Inverness or Glasgow. But at the same time there is a greater expectation of what medicine could or should do and a greater readiness to call the doctor for problems that would in the past have been unrecognized or tolerated, according to the stoicism that was once the dominant characteristic of Hebridean health culture.

When John Robertson took up his post in Tarbert twenty years ago house calls were a rarity. 'Stoicism was one reason, but there were others – self-sufficiency, politeness. Gaelic people are very polite and don't like to bother the doctor. And there was and still is a different attitude to time; if something isn't done today, it can be done tomorrow. There's no urgency and that applies to calling a GP as well as everything else.'

Attitudes are changing, particularly among the young, or at least those of them who stay, and to doctors who have worked for years in island communities, this has had a noticeable impact on health care. But even more important has been the shift in population age, which has shaped the illnesses of the Hebrides as much as it has moulded the appearance of villages and the residential needs of those who live in them. The Western Isles have a reputation for heart disease, even more than Scotland as a whole. And Scotland has the highest rate in the world.

High blood pressure may be one explanation. It is common in older people everywhere but there is a belief among doctors that on the islands it is more widespread than it should be, even after the age of the people is taken into account. Because it is usually linked to heart disease it could contribute to the numerous cases arising in the Isles. Yet there is research to suggest that the Hebrideans are relatively protected from the usual impact of raised blood pressure on the heart. The signs of heart strain shown up by electrocardiogram are less than would be expected from the measured pressure. So, although there is plenty of heart disease, there is less of it than there should be.

John Robertson believed in the protection theory. Perhaps increased vulnerability may even encourage a population to develop its own natural protection. He was equally sure that both heart disease and hypertension could be attributed in part to the Hebridean way of life. Although heredity and smoking shared the blame, it was in the island diet that he saw the most specific risks. 'People here eat salty herring and salty meat, both beef and mutton. They make puddings out of seaweed. The diet is full of salt and cholesterol. And there is a lot of obesity.'

He believed in another twist in medical logic too: that despite suffering the worst rate of the country's biggest cause of death, the people of the Outer Hebrides live longer. There were many families whose members aged over eighty were all fit and active. Perhaps the outdoor life kept people healthy. But once again he emphasized the low stress, the lack of urgency in the culture – not simple procrastination, which carries a connotation of wasting time, but an acceptance that where the sea and the weather are unpredictable and the land treacherous, tomorrow might well be better than today.

Back at the hotel I began to learn the same lesson. Isadora was now blustering at her peak and was not expected to relax for twenty-four hours. The next morning's ferry had after all been cancelled and the hotel staff were not only acting as if they had predicted the delay all along, but were now hinting that I might be marooned for days. There was, I realized, no contradiction in their change of mind because in one sense going and not going meant the same thing: to them it simply didn't matter. To me it did; as soon as I discovered I was stuck there I was desperate to leave.

By evening the hotel bar had become a sanctuary from the storm. Streams and even streets were gushing. To go outside was to be pelted and drenched. Stranded visitors to Harris bought drinks for the locals as if appeasing some angry Hebridean god and anxiously eyed the weather reports which brought only bad news. They also confirmed that the amateur auguries had been right: the wind was only force eleven which for some reason I was mildly disappointed to hear.

Even by the following morning there had been no let-up in the storm. Like the Eskimos with their numerous words for snow covering all its varieties, the Hebrideans must have countless words for cold and wet. Not wanting to spend the day cooped up, I took a tour of the south part of Harris, an excursion Halliday Sutherland undertook by a bus that he thought was too battered to complete the trip. As he travelled he mused on why men who invest money in the Hebrides, James Matheson included, end up losing it.

Harris looks like nowhere else I have ever seen. It is completely unlike the Scottish mainland with its tourist-trapping blend of mountains and lochs. But it also looks nothing like Shetland, though both are made of moors and cliffs, or even Skye with its jagged mountain contour. More than anything Harris resembles a bad film set designed to conjure up an alien planet. It is a mound of glacial rock and sodden peat, littered with huge boulders and heavily scattered with patches of black moorland water too numerous and untidy to be called lakes. There is hardly a tree standing; supposedly in 1098, during the days of Norwegian rule, one Magnus Bareleg burned them all.

But some of its coast is as striking as any slice of Cornwall and only its mist and rain keep the superlatives in check. Where the road meets the broad sand plains at Horgabost on its north-west shoulder I tried to look across the sea to the island of Taransay and thought I could make out its silhouette through the haze. When the crofters on Taransay wanted Dr Robertson to visit, they used to send one of their boats to this stretch of coast to pick him up. Crofting brought its own diseases, mainly infections caught from sheep, but these are not common now that crofting is in decline and the Tarbert practice no longer has patients on the island.

People have gone too from Pabbay, another chunk of rock off the Harris shoreline, reputedly emptied forcibly because of its illegal still. In fact there is surprisingly little talk of illegal whisky on Harris compared to some islands around the Scottish coast, and no legal distillery to rival those on the larger inner isles. The Hebrideans, despite sharing the highland reputation for drink, have always been able to defend their honour with superficial estimates of how much they consume. In the mid-nineteenth century, for instance, when both urban and rural Scotland abounded in whisky dens, the Western Isles possessed fewer than any other region. Yet the impression of heavy consumption sticks, as it always does wherever spirits are drunk alongside temperance.

As with blood pressure and the heart, there is a unique island paradox to the medical impact of the whisky dram. Doctors here have found less liver cirrhosis than the overall consumption would suggest and, to popular acclaim, have attributed this happy circumstance to the 'fact' that whisky is less poisonous to the liver than other alcoholic drinks.

Beyond the southern end of Harris, past the point that overlooked Pabbay, the road grew thinner and more winding. Great pools gathered at the roadsides and minor torrents from the hills poured across the tarmac. All this surface liquid and thick sheets of rain made me feel I was steadily being engulfed by water. And there was something else that enhanced the weird ambience: every few miles I passed wrecked cars abandoned months or years ago to rot amongst the bracken. They made a strange sight and, added to the general bleakness, conjured up a different sort of desolation, as if I had dropped in for the afternoon on some post-holocaust world.

Such distant depopulated parts of the planet are said to provide protection to those who, in becoming psychotic, develop feelings of fear and threat. It has been claimed that schizophrenia is prevalent in the Hebrides as well as in the similarly deserted territory of northern Scandinavia, perhaps because the conditions are more acceptable to someone who finds a human environment disturbing. So the usual pattern of higher rates of mental illness in migrants, crucial to the controversy over mental illness in Bristol, is reversed. According to one theory, the comparatively immune, upwardly mobile islanders head for mainland cities and by doing so raise the proportion of island residents who will develop schizophrenia. Those who do become ill find the empty space to their liking and stay. But the truth is that no one knows the reason for the excess. Indeed the rate may not be high at all, if John Robertson's experience is typical. Among the 2,000 people on his list, ten have schizophrenia, half what the general population rate would predict.

Despite the talk of low environmental stress, there is no reason to be starry-eyed about the traditional life in these islands. They may have escaped the deadlines of urban living but they are generously endowed with the equivalent stresses of physical hardship, as the occasional settler from the mainland discovers. The native Hebrideans talk of these immigrants with a sympathetic mockery: they come here hoping to find peace and purity, they say, intending to polish shells and live off the sea. But they don't stay. Even John Robertson talked of leaving, as if he was planning the final stage of his career, though he was young enough for it to run for nearly twenty more years.

Later, in the early evening, refreshed by the news that my ferry would be sailing at five the next morning – the hotel staff claimed to have expected this as well – I followed the north road out of Tarbert along the rim of the West Loch and between towering mountains with unpronounceable Gaelic names. The sky had cleared but the moors themselves were dark as if the two had lost their synchrony. Until the road began to climb, the wind felt like no more than the final swish of Isadora's skirt but nearer the summits it threatened to send me veering into the roadside rocks. At one time the journey through these peaks was so slow and unpleasant that travellers between Lewis and Harris went by sea, creating the myth that they are separate islands.

Towards the end of his journey Halliday Sutherland came to sound like a man brooding more and more on his life's course, gently complaining of declining fitness, which he saw as the first intrusion of mortality. When in his closing pages he was landed at the Kyle of Lochalsh by a trawler, he looked back at the Western Isles and saw them in a metaphorical sleep not unlike the eternal one he felt he was turning to face. But the grave, self-deprecating manner was all nonsense. Halliday lived well into his seventies, 'the most cocksure man in the British Empire', as Marie Stopes described him, shortly before he sued her for some other libel.

Something about these islands turns people like Halliday pensive and melancholy: the harshness of the climate, I was ready to believe, but something else as well, affecting visitors and even non-native residents, because unlike religion or a taste for whisky, being Hebridean cannot be developed by practice. Being an outsider here is a permanent state and a naturally sombre one.

I too left in sober mood. The trouble with scratching the surface, as I had done to the culture of the Western Isles, is that you don't know how much surface is left. The island reputation for booze and the Bible now seemed not simply wrong but grotesque, most of all where medicine was concerned. Whisky, it had turned out, was popular but surprisingly non-toxic and Free Presbyterianism was positively healthy. Yet just as there were contradictions to be found by peeling away the surface image so there must have been further twists lying below the undersurface which would in turn challenge my impression if only I was familiar enough with the Hebrides to see them. And even then, how could I be sure that I had seen Harris clearly? However aware of the place I might become, there would always be a sense that something was hidden.

But I was certain of one thing. Hebridean tradition is being irreversibly dismantled by economic progress – new roads, the departure of young people, the demand for gadgets – and medicine is not only feeling the changes but dominated by them. The insularity which has held the islands together and frustrated all-comers is now cracking from the inside.

EIGHT

Edinburgh

IF THE appearance of a city centre is a clue to its character, then Edinburgh has its dark side. Although the area is crowded with majestic, ancient buildings, there are dingy alleys slotted between them: short cuts, tradesmen's closes and paths to tenement entrances and public houses. It is a city approaching old age, famous in Scotland for its stiff air of disapproval, the only place in the country that would call its Georgian quarter the New Town, with a skill that goes with old age, the ability to brag about its history and conceal the truth about what it has really been up to.

Edinburgh's medicine is equally rooted in the past, in the eighteenth and nineteenth centuries when its teaching was unrivalled. Most of the great doctors of the period passed through the medical school or its main hospital, and new ideas in pain relief and the control of infection flourished. The city's medical history is packed with pomp and incident, towering characters and great thoughts. But it too has its dark side.

My initial aim was to look around the collection of hospital buildings on Lauriston Place, still dominated by the original Infirmary, and now expanded by modern blocks of laboratories and clinics. The front entrance to the hospital is forbidden to medical students, in keeping with the city's stuffy reputation, less a product of snobbery than of fuddy-duddery. Inside the names of benefactors are listed on the walls, including that of David Hume. But the name that interested me most was on the dull block at the back of the Royal Infirmary complex. This was the maternity hospital – or pavilion, as it is quaintly called – and the name it celebrates is Sir James Young Simpson, who not only revolutionized surgery by introducing chloroform as an anaesthetic but also turned the care of pregnant women into something respectable.

The foundations to Simpson's pavilion were laid a hundred years or so after he graduated from the medical school in 1832 at the age of twenty-one. Unlike many doctors of the day his background was distinctly ordinary, without any hint of the high society that would later patronize him. He was the seventh child of a baker in Bathgate, eighteen miles west of Edinburgh, a town that had produced no one else of renown in the 500 years since one of its dignitaries had married Robert the Bruce's daughter. Simpson left Bathgate to live in the capital at the age of fourteen and after two unsettled years he enrolled as a medical student in 1827.

Part of the training was to observe leading surgeons at work which, as it was carried out without anaesthesia, was a gruesome business. The Edinburgh doctor and short story writer John Brown described in *Rab and his Friends* how his classmates burst into tears after watching a woman being held down for an operation. One of Simpson's student contemporaries, Charles Darwin, ran out of two operations, refused to go back and eventually gave up medicine. Simpson himself is reported to have left the theatre during a breast amputation by Liston, one of Edinburgh's surgical chiefs, because he could not bear the look of horror on the patient's face.

It was also Liston who, by his use of ether some years later, awakened Simpson to the medical value of gases, something which Thomas Beddoes of Bristol and his assistant Humphry Davy could have told them about long before (in fact it was Davy's own protégé Michael Faraday who discovered that ether could be used as an anaesthetic). The advantage of ether was not just that it relieved the patient's pain. It also allowed the surgeon to cut more quickly and accurately and so reduced the extent of trauma and the risk of death. Along with Joseph Lister of antisepsis fame, Simpson attended a demonstration in which Liston amputated the leg of his anaesthetized patient, a butler called Frederick Churchill, in no more than twenty-eight seconds. He was impressed and immediately introduced ether into his own practice.

By now Simpson was well established in Edinburgh medicine but in a fairly disreputable branch of the profession, midwifery. Childbirth took place at home and it was partly this that prompted him to look for his own anaesthetic vapour. The large glass bottles in which ether had to be carried around were too heavy to lug up the stairs of tenements. In addition, his well-to-do patients, who were also his own neighbours in the New Town, complained of the smell of ether which tended to linger long after its use.

Simpson and his acolytes set about finding a substitute by sniffing a variety of laboratory chemicals but, as often happens in science, the successful discovery did not originate with the man who became known for it. It was an Edinburgh chemist called David Waldie who suggested chloroform, a newly-described liquid giving off a vapour that had been shown to render animals unconscious. But Simpson dismissed it on the not unreasonable grounds that the animals had then died. Waldie planned to prove Simpson wrong and sent to London for a supply of chloroform, but it never arrived.

Only when his assistant Matthews Duncan, who was by now the veteran of many a sniffing experiment covering acetone, iodine and various other substances, expressed optimism about chloroform did Simpson reconsider. In a memorable evening in his home in Queen Street he, Duncan and a third man called Dr Keith inhaled it and thus discovered its effects. Initially the three men became over-talkative and supposedly entertained the ladies present, but a short time thereafter they were deeply asleep.

Soon after, on 9 November 1847, chloroform was put through its first clinical trial. The patient, Jane Carstairs, the wife of a doctor, was in her second pregnancy, her first child having died after a painful labour lasting more than three days. Three hours into this labour, Simpson poured half a teaspoonful of chloroform liquid on to a handkerchief and placed it over her face. Within twenty-five minutes he had delivered the baby. When its mother woke up she at first refused to believe that the child could be hers.

The use of the new gas to abolish the pain of childbirth drew criticism for being unnatural – the same charge that had been made against vaccination – and for contravening the biblical edict that children should be brought forth in sorrow. But Simpson was a persuasive advocate and chloroform was soon reducing mortality from many types of surgery. By 1850 it had been used in almost 100,000 cases in Edinburgh alone. When three years later it was given to Queen Victoria as she delivered her eighth child, Leopold, its success was established.

Simpson became a celebrity beyond medical circles and was courted by the artists and literati of the day. His daughter went skating with the young Robert Louis Stevenson; and John Ruskin, who was said to admire Simpson for his knowledge of sperm whales, arranged a consultation for his unhappy wife Effie Gray. Being an obstetrician Simpson concluded that Effie needed a few children, a view that was discussed in court when the marriage was famously annulled on grounds of non-consummation and impotence.

Across Middle Meadow Walk from the Infirmary stands the medical school, the descendant of the school of anatomy that brought students to Edinburgh from the mid-eighteenth century onwards, and now part of the university complex. Although Simpson's story embodies all the characteristics of an Edinburgh medical triumph, there have been other routes to prominence for men who studied here. Not everyone appreciated the education on offer; some were quick to look elsewhere for their vocation. Darwin was one of these: unable to watch operations, bored by anatomy and scathing about the Royal Medical Society where he said 'much rubbish was talked', he spent his time stuffing birds and trawling for oysters with fishermen from the port of Newhaven.

Oliver Goldsmith was another example. Hampered by what is sometimes referred to as his artistic temperament, he attended only anatomy classes, telling a friend that 'an hereditary indolence' kept him away from all other study, although it did not stop him from dancing jigs for the amusement of the local aristocracy. Eventually he left Edinburgh intending to train in France but on the voyage was taken ashore and imprisoned as a spy – a lucky mistake as the ship he had been on subsequently sank (or so he claimed).

But of all the doctors who passed through the anatomy school none is better known than Joseph Bell, though his distinction was achieved not as himself but through his fictional alter ego, Sherlock Holmes. After graduating from Edinburgh in 1859, Bell became a demonstrator in anatomy and was later an assistant to the Queen's surgeon Patrick Heron Watson. Despite the failure of his application for Edinburgh's top surgical job – Joseph Lister beat him to it – he became the most skilful teacher of the period, and the most popular with students, of whom Conan Doyle was one.

Bell was an irrepressible show-off. His teaching technique was to conduct his first interview with patients in front of a full lecture theatre, mesmerizing his students with a combination of brilliant observation and good guesswork. It was a time when ordinary people spent their lives pursuing a particular trade which might leave its mark on them, in the stain of a factory dye or the smell of an animal. Some jobs would gradually induce a tell-tale posture, others would affect the roughness of the hands or the colour of the complexion. Many led to specific diseases.

It was this that allowed Bell to preach that keen observation was the key to good medicine and to practise his creed so flamboyantly, making deductions about his patients that went way beyond diagnosis. One illustrative account has him demonstrating his ability on a young woman, admitted to his presence carrying an infant. After an exchange of greetings, Bell fired at her the following four questions: Had she had a good crossing from Burntisland? Had she enjoyed her walk up Inverleith Row? What had she done with her other child? Did she still work in a linoleum factory? If his students were fascinated, his patient must have been bewildered. But it was all in the observation: her first words had revealed a Fife accent and Burntisland was the nearest Fife town where she would have been able to board a boat to Edinburgh. Inverleith Row was a likely route for her walk from the shore and the red clay on her shoes confirmed it. The coat she was carrying was too big for the child on her arm and the inflammation of her right hand was probably a contact dermatitis acquired in Burntisland's linoleum factory. Elementary.

Patients corrected his conclusions at their peril, as shown by one incident which Bell himself recorded. As soon as that morning's case was ushered in, before the man had even spoken, Bell announced that he played the bagpipes in a Highland regiment, explaining to the audience that his posture and his short stature placed him in a military band while his swaggering gait was typical of a piper. But the man spoiled the show by denying that he had ever been in the army and insisting that he was a shoemaker. Bell's confidence in his own powers – not to mention what doctors could get away with – must have been considerable because he had his patient removed to another room and stripped. On the luckless piper's chest was printed an indelible blue 'D', the sign of what he had hoped to conceal, his desertion in Crimea.

Conan Doyle made no secret of the fact that Bell was his model for Holmes and the surgeon was much in demand as a public figure. He even engaged in forensic work and used his sharp eye not just to describe medical evidence but to relate it to clues from the scene of a crime. At times it must have seemed that Bell was beginning to be based on Holmes, not the other way round, especially when, as is supposed to have happened, one convicted murderer, about to be hanged, asserted that he would have escaped had it not been for the doctor's testimony. And there is a story which, if true, could have made Bell the greatest of detectives. In 1888 he took a deep interest in London's Ripper murders and having investigated the details he is said to have notified Edinburgh's *Scotsman* newspaper of the killer's identity. But, as Sherlock Holmes often found, the authorities were sceptical of his genius and the revelation never made it into print.

A short way along Forest Road from the medical school is the entrance to Greyfriars churchyard, a proximity that must have been useful in the days when grave-robbing to supply the dissecting tables was a thriving industry. A lot has been written about Burke and Hare, who sold their murdered victims to teachers of anatomy, and of the complicity of Robert Knox, the doctor whom an Edinburgh song of the time described as 'the man who buys the beef'. But the context of their activities is less often exposed.

Even before the first school of anatomy opened in Edinburgh in the early eighteenth century, a hundred years before Knox arrived in the capital, bodies were being stolen from Greyfriars cemetery by surgeons' apprentices and used as a means of learning. The city's College of Surgeons acknowledged as much in 1711 and as a result it was written into the terms of employment of apprentices that they were forbidden from violating churchyards. Not that this made any difference and by 1725 public outrage had reached such a pitch that the anatomy school was fortunate not to have been torn down.

As Edinburgh's teaching reputation grew, so did the demand for cadavers. No longer was body-snatching merely a sideline for apprentices and gravediggers, it was now a career in itself. Bribes were passed and, time being money, corpses were often removed *before* burial with the help of sextons and mourners. So skilled were the Edinburgh resurrectionists that by the turn of the century there was an export trade to London, the unusual cargo being surreptitiously shipped out of Leith in boxes marked 'perishable goods'.

The reaction of the public was ambivalent; people were against the desecration of graves as sinful but many recognized that the end result was a better qualified medical profession, from which they might benefit. Similarly the fact that the law was on the look-out for suspicious visitors to the anatomy rooms ignored the point that the students themselves were sometimes part of the illegal business. But because it was illegal and therefore clandestine it always took place within Edinburgh's underworld, a natural arena for additional criminal activity, and mutual swindling was a common feature of body-snatching deals. It was inevitable that it would sooner or later occur to someone that murder was a good way of lubricating the market.

Down the slope of Candlemaker Row I came to the Grassmarket, the open confluence of five roads, where many city trades were once concentrated. With the Castle looming on one side and a tall row of grime-stained buildings on the other, it provides a suitable setting for Edinburgh's low-life and, although it is now a favourite spot for young people to drink al fresco, its name until not many years ago was synonymous with alcoholic homelessness. In the early nineteenth century it was the scene of heavy drinking, prostitution and crime.

William Hare and his wife ran a lodging house in Tanner's Close, off the West Port, another of the routes down to the Grassmarket, and William Burke occupied one of his rooms. When in November 1827 another lodger died owing Hare £4 in rent, he and Burke came up with the idea of selling the man's body to recover the loss. They therefore filled his coffin with bark from the tanner's yard outside their home and carried the corpse to the anatomy school. There a medical student redirected them to Robert Knox's private demonstration rooms; without this chance intervention Knox might never have been involved.

Burke and Hare were paid £7.10s for their specimen, a tempting profit. Shortly afterwards, when another of Hare's lodgers took sick, the two men chose to smother him rather than run the risk that he might recover. Over the next year they killed fifteen others, mainly prostitutes and solitary individuals whom they lured to their home, plied with drink and asphyxiated. This method of killing left no tell-tale mark of injury and allowed them to claim to Knox and his assistants that the victims had died of internal illness, such as might be caused by alcohol. Although dissection should have revealed to the anatomists that there was no liver disease, infection or other pathological change, no suspicion was voiced until a medical student recognized one of the corpses as a Grassmarket prostitute, Mary Paterson. But Burke insisted she too had died of drink and that he had bought her from 'an old hag' in Canongate, a street nearby.

Only after two tenants at Hare's lodging house had seen a woman's body under some straw were the murderers caught – unlike doctors, lodgers were one group of people with an unambiguous interest in ending the trade – but even this victim was in Knox's cellar by the time the law arrived. Charges of wilful murder were brought against Hare, Hare's wife, Burke and Helen McDougal, Burke's mistress. But at the trial on Christmas Eve 1828 the Hares turned King's evidence and were freed to return to their native Ireland. Burke, however, was not only hanged but publicly dissected, though not by Knox. That task fell to the medical school's leading anatomist, Professor Munro, the man to whom Burke and Hare had hoped to sell their first corpse until a student redirected them to Knox. The case against McDougal was 'not proven'.

The citizens of Edinburgh were horrified and fascinated by the crime and took the chance to see Burke receive his just desert. Twenty thousand turned out in pouring rain to watch him hang at the corner of the High Street above the Grassmarket and seats with a clear view were sold for twenty-five shillings to the well off, possibly including Sir Walter Scott. So many crammed into the dissection room afterwards that medical students were unable to squeeze in. Yet the opportunity for popular revenge was limited by the escape from punishment of three of the four accused and this may have fuelled the subsequent outcry against Knox.

But had he known what Burke and Hare were up to? The Edinburgh mob were in no doubt and made an attempt to lynch him, although the closest they came was to hang his effigy. But more sober voices also spoke against him, including the Church and some of his own profession. Sir Walter Scott believed that 'five or six others', Knox among them, were just as guilty as Burke.

Knox himself made matters worse by initially refusing to say anything about the affair, foolishly hoping that it would blow over, but as the attacks on his character increased he was forced to write to the *Caledonian Chronicle* to declare his innocence. Finally a committee of distinguished persons investigated his role in the crime and accused him only of being 'incautious' in the way he had bought bodies. It did, however, refer to the absence of any sign of illness on the fresh corpses he purchased and to the unconvincing explanations given by Burke. Though he eventually resigned and moved to London he was never able to shake off the taint of notoriety. The next few years were made more miserable by the death of his wife and son and a further scandal concerning a bogus physician, who possessed certificates of attendance at his lectures.

In one way Knox was himself a victim: of the body-snatching that was long established when he came to Edinburgh, which many dissecting rooms had welcomed and over which city officials had been complacent. It took the Burke and Hare outrage and another case in London before Parliament set down rules on the donation of corpses to licensed dissectors, rules that would take the process out of the hands of profiteers and criminals generally. But if the question of his personal guilt comes down to whether he was naïve about Burke and Hare or chose to ignore what he preferred not to believe, it has to be admitted that no one ever accused him of *naïveté* over anything else. James Bridie, a doctor as well as a playwright, portrayed him as entertaining but arrogant; as a lecturer his flamboyant brilliance was said to be admired by students (Simpson was one) but despised by colleagues. Born into a family that claimed kinship with John Knox, the Presbyterian reformer, he was a worldly man who served as an army surgeon at Waterloo and later practised at the Cape of Good Hope where he wrote authoritatively on many subjects, medical and otherwise. One of these was the behaviour of hyenas, from whose habit of living off dead flesh he should perhaps have learned more.

The road from the centre of town dipped downhill to Canonmills and along Inverleith Row, still the likeliest route to the coast, as it was in Bell's day, and then further north to where it hooked round to Granton Harbour. The Firth of Forth was dotted with sails as the local yachting fraternity took advantage of the bright afternoon; this was the well-heeled version of Edinburgh, able to look across its own estuary to the Fife hills, a city without an inner city, but up Granton Road lay its dark side, one of Britain's ugliest estates and the scene of one of the most urgent of its health problems.

Across an old railway bridge were the housing blocks that mark the beginning of Pilton, not so much high-rise as long-stretch because they continued at a height of three or four storeys as far west as I could see. Parking my car on the main road, I walked back to the buildings known as West Granton View and West Granton Gardens. Needless to say, however, this is virtually the only point along the city's northern highways where there is no view, except of the gasworks that blocks the outlook over the Forth, and the only gardens are a patch of waste land.

This part of Pilton looks like a ghost town and I half-expected to see tumbleweed blowing towards me across the concrete. Most of it is boarded up. Only about one in ten of the windows shows any sign of life inside and only the odd balcony is strung with washing. The walls are filthy and their numerous cracks have been cemented over in a way that makes them more obvious. In fact, so striking are they that from a distance they give the impression of being an unusual mosaic, though certainly one that has gone wrong. The conventional form of urban art, graffiti, is abundant, though largely mysterious, much of it consisting of words and symbols I couldn't decipher. The rest reports on the details of local romances but there is one wall where someone with an ironic sense of humour has painted what appear to be sunflowers and another that sports the words EAT THE RICH.

Becoming a general practitioner in this area would not be most people's idea of a good career move but Pilton has led Roy Robertson to carry out influential research, and to become prominent enough for his opinions to invite criticism in the press. Yet his move into sensitive areas of medical practice happened almost by accident; medicine will often pull a person from one topic to another as the complexity of their chosen subject becomes apparent. In Dr Robertson's case the starting point was the physical abuse of children which, as a newly qualified GP, he felt was rife in the run-down estates where his practice is based. Abuse was then big news in medicine and much public concern had been aroused. But it was soon clear that in Pilton and the neighbouring district of Muirhouse it was only one aspect of a social and medical crisis at the centre of which was poverty. Another manifestation of the same thing was the widespread use of heroin, so from his interest in the safety of Pilton's children Roy Robertson moved into the problems of drug addiction, and from there he began to study Aids.

Over the expanse of waste ground were rows of houses rather than flats and I headed for these in the approximate direction of Roy's surgery. Apart from one teenager with a pram the open field was deserted until a biker in leather gear surprised me by bursting out of one of the doorways in West Granton View. Around the fringes of what was presumably meant to be parkland were piles of rubbish, some of it recently incinerated, and scattered detritus that was currently drawing the attention of one or two overblown dogs. There were torn paper sacks, there was shattered glass, and even one of the lampposts was in pieces.

Before long I was drawing unwelcoming looks from the doorways, long questioning gazes that followed my progress along each street. That outsiders were easy to spot I had no doubt, and that many signified trouble of one sort or another was not hard to imagine. Passing through a gap in a fence I skirted round a school and reached a plot of threadbare grass which claimed to be a recreation area – empty, of course.

In the first wave of concern over drugs in Pilton in the early 1980s, it was said that schools had become a thriving market for the pushers, that bored adolescents heading for unemployment could buy heroin at school gates. Roy Robertson can remember little evidence of any such scene. It may have happened, he told me, but he did not see it. Yet undoubtedly there had been a change in the pattern of drug use. At the beginning of the 1970s Edinburgh's drug culture was limited both geographically and chemically, being concentrated in the city centre and more or less confined to cannabis and pharmaceutical substances. But as time went by there was a shift towards intravenous drugs, including heroin. Simultaneously the number of people buying such substances multiplied as supplies were brought from London and sold in centrally located pubs.

What happened next was critical to the subsequent spread of HIV. 'Around 1979 to 1980, large quantites of heroin flooded the market from some eastern countries,' Roy Robertson recalled, 'and there was a rapid expansion in the number of people injecting. They were different from what we had seen before. They were younger, there were more women and they lived on the periphery of the city in the poor housing estates. In the next few years heroin was common in this area. There were several houses round here where you could buy it. There was even a letter box that you put money in and heroin was handed out. You didn't have to say anything.'

When Roy surveyed the intravenous heroin users listed with his practice, he found most to be in their early twenties but threequarters of them had started in their teens, usually after being introduced to the drug by a friend. Most had no job but were spending between £5 and £150 per day on their habit. About half had suffered illnesses related to drug-taking – either infections or jaundice, a sign of hepatitis – and it was this that proved the most ominous of his findings. It indicated poor hygiene and the shared use of dirty equipment. In fact almost two-thirds of those who took part in the study, all of whom were injecting daily, admitted to sharing needles.

Such a young population of users, largely ignorant of the medical dangers they were exposing themselves to, and certainly careless of the risks of passing around their apparatus, was highly susceptible to the as yet unrecognized spread of HIV, but other circumstances also conspired to make its transmission easier.

First, there was an emphasis on tackling drugs through legal controls and specifically through heavy penalties for those found guilty of drug offences, with the result that the therapeutic needs of the young addict appeared less important. Arrests increased and long gaol terms were dished out to those caught in possession of fairly small amounts of heroin. Scotland's legal authorities took the view that by punishing the ordinary user, the end point in the chain of supply, they would move nearer to the bigger fish further up the chain. Whether or not deterrent sentencing was successful in reducing drug use – and there are those who would argue that it was – the debate over Edinburgh's drug problem was now focused on crime and retribution. The press, picking up the prevalent political line, referred to anti-drug measures as a war. 'The police often stated that 50 per cent of housebreaking was drug-related,' said Roy, 'so I traced back this statement to find out where the figure came from. It was just a policeman's opinion. Anyway, what does drug-related mean? If your partner is taking drugs and you burgle somebody, does that count as drug-related? The figure didn't mean anything.' Not unlike the supply of bodies for dissection, the trade in heroin responded to legal restriction by submerging itself in an illicit underworld, increasingly out of reach of any services that might coax individuals away from their addiction.

Second, the services themselves were experiencing a period of disillusionment and regular contact with the growing number of young users was proving hard to maintain. In any case those who had recently begun injecting were still enjoying it and saw no need for help. Many who did want to give up did not find the hospital-based treatment to their liking and in turn the doctors running the service became pessimistic about what they had to offer. Committee-room discussions and reports followed, eventually leading to a new approach to drug dependence in Pilton, one that combined medical and social care in a community setting. But it all took time and for much of the early 1980s the people working on the problem were struggling to contain it.

Then there was the fact that a lack of clean equipment for injection made it more likely that needles and syringes would be passed around. The shortage was no accident. It was the recommendation of pharmaceutical authorities that no such apparatus should be available; one retailer who continued to sell it went out of business after some local doctors withdrew their custom and after there was pressure from the police to stop selling it. The argument – that making fresh needles scarce would force addicts to give up – now sounds specious. But its opposite, that distributing needles to drug users would help control hepatitis, seemed eccentric, out of step with the philosophy of the day. Only later did it emerge that the risk did not end with hepatitis.

Past a dentist's surgery that was so fortified against theft that it looked like a pillbox, I reached Roy's practice, its external design reflecting the style, if that is the right word, of the surrounding estates. Inside it was different: surrounded by a bank of computers his research team was studying the pattern of HIV infection in Pilton and Muirhouse. In 1985 it was found that the virus had penetrated Edinburgh's drug-injecting population and, collaborating with virologists and public health physicians, Roy Robertson studied its prevalence in blood samples taken from local drug-users and stored since 1982, when there had been an outbreak of hepatitis. The results were dramatic: 51 per cent were found to be infected but the true rate was thought to be much higher because some of the negative samples were not recent. Edinburgh had been shown to have the most serious HIV epidemic in Britain; this reservoir of infection among heterosexuals meant that the potential for spread was unlimited.

Most of those who had caught the virus were thought to have done so between 1983 and 1985 and though many factors must have been responsible, needle sharing was at the heart of the matter. The case for needle exchange schemes was now compelling but still there was opposition. Roy remembered raising the subject while speaking at a conference: 'I said needles should be given out to prevent sharing. One newspaper present rang the police and asked if this was legal. The police said they didn't know, they would have to check with their medical lawyers. But the next day the paper said the police had told me that it was illegal and printed a photo of me looking as if I'd been caught doing something wrong, with a huge headline, DR ROBERTSON WARNED.'

Professional groups such as doctors and pharmacists were against it and the Edinburgh police opposed it, saying that it broke laws on the supply of drug-taking equipment. Senior judges in Scotland confirmed that exchanging new needles for old was illegal. But a change was inevitable, though the 1987 pilot schemes too ran into trouble when local residents picketed them. Even some drug users were initially suspicious, fearing that they would be watched by the law. Since then pick-up points for fresh needles have proliferated and now include GP surgeries where scepticism was once strong. There is even a bus run by the city's Health Board to make needles and condoms more accessible.

Combined with a campaign of education, the schemes appear to have had some effect. When in 1990 Roy studied the drug users whom he had not identified until after the first alarm over HIV in 1985, he found the rate of infection to have fallen to 29 per cent; this is still disturbingly high, proving that even the threat of Aids, like the threat of hepatitis before it, is insufficient to deter users from dirty injecting, contrary to the belief held by those who opposed needle exchange.

Among the older addicts, those who started as teenagers in the early 1980s, the pattern of drug-taking has evolved: towards new drugs, also administered intravenously, and intermittent use, prompted by the restricted availability of heroin, the prospect of stern punishment and, for some, enforced absence from the scene through imprisonment. Another influence has been the passage of time, the effect of the 'maturing subculture' as it is styled. Many ex-addicts have families, a few are in work. Groups of friends have grown apart, diminishing the communal shooting-up sessions that were once popular and where contaminated equipment was easily borrowed. Roy's research shows that one in twelve has died, though only a minority from Aids.

Almost two-thirds of his patients who were known to be injecting before the mid-1980s are now HIV positive. This is an appalling figure in itself but there is a further menace in what it heralds for others. In these older users the rate of HIV infection, if not quite stable, is no longer accelerating. In their younger counterparts the prevalence is lower, even on follow-up tests. But the extent to which the virus has passed into the general population of young adults is uncertain and, because of the long incubation period of Aids, will remain unquantifiable unless there are repeated surveys substantial enough to provide a reliable answer, a massive – not to mention controversial – task.

The evidence from high-risk areas such as Pilton, where preliminary findings point to an infection rate among young adults of one in fourteen for men and one in twenty-eight for women, predict disaster. Unless transmission is controlled, heterosexual sex will replace intravenous drug use as its main vehicle, as in those parts of Africa where infection is similarly endemic, and the numbers harbouring the disease will become overwhelming. But how to control it?

From Roy Robertson's perspective, the most important measures are those that will take place on the ground where the risks are greatest, as was true of the treatment of addicts, and he does not approve of the fact that most money for research on HIV goes into hospitals. Edinburgh's Aids crisis is happening in his practice, in people's homes, to families, to young mothers, to dejected adolescents. Those who inject have to be taught to do so safely. Unprotected sex has to be convincingly discouraged. 'At one extreme, you could say we have to have large studies to prevent the future epidemic, to save us from destruction. At the other you could say: who are these researchers who are bothering these poor folk? We're in the community, trying to tread a middle line.'

On my way back to my car I passed two families sitting outside their neighbouring ground-floor flats, the adults relaxing, the children not quite fighting. They were living in the middle of the most frightening of diseases, one that was probably spreading, invisibly and therefore more dangerously. They were at the centre of what could become the biggest public health catastrophe for decades. Were they terrified? Or was Aids just another blow on a long list that included lack of money, jobs and decent housing?

I drove up Pennywell Road, a broad featureless carriageway separating Pilton from Muirhouse, overlooked by the Muirhouse surgery, and at a roundabout at the far corner of the district, I turned towards the city centre again, travelling through Edinburgh's better-known scenery. A row of bungalows here, a posh school there, it looked like a different world.

NINE

Scarborough

IF IT was a typical year, I was one of 2 million visitors to Scarborough, most of us crammed into a few summer months, each looking for our own version of a good time. If it was a typical bank holiday, I would need luck to find somewhere to stay that night. But from early in the day when I had seen my car heat up and break down on the way here, I had had the feeling that my luck was out. Time would tell.

A trip to a holiday resort is a kind of pilgrimage. It begins with an arduous journey, leads to an immersion in water if only up to the ankles, and ends with the belief that it has all been worth it; someone who travels for the sake of his health will never admit to disappointment. But towns like Scarborough know how unhealthy holidays can be. When the tourist season begins, they have to absorb an overnight tripling of their population, an influx that threatens to engulf hospitals and ambulances designed to cater only for the locals. This mass of migrants may be bent on pleasure and fitness but in seeking it they fall ill. They break their bones, strain their backs, lose their pills, forget their age, drink too much beer, eat the wrong food, fight, fall and jaywalk.

When they do, they end up where I was now arriving, the Casualty block of Scarborough Hospital, on the outer border of the town; perhaps it should have been built high up beside the castle between the two bays, as a warning to the bathers on the beaches below. Between Whitsun and early October this hospital department is stretched and at times overwhelmed by visitors to the town. During these months three-quarters of its patients are in the area on vacation. When I reached the waiting area, however, its rows of chairs were deserted and the staff were in a back room taking a protracted break.

Casualty staff the world over are the same. They have seen every-thing and are unshockable. They love to astonish their audiences with tales of the indelicate trauma that can befall their fellow humans, or lurid accounts of the retribution that awaits those who break the laws of natural behaviour. As a result their stories of life at the sharp end of health care are often about sex, newly-weds and lavatories, like picture postcards from a seaside resort, the sort you can buy on the Scar-borough sea front.

The Casualty nurses I met entertained me with many such anec-dotes, some of them strikingly similar to others I had heard in the past and elsewhere, before they spoke of the season's chief crisis so far: jellyfish. There was a plague of them round the two bays and hapless bathers were being brought in daily. 'One boy came in with a jellyfish still attached to his leg,' Chris Hughes, sister in charge, told me in a tale reminiscent of the bedroom light-bulb stories I had recently been listening to.

If the jellyfish didn't get you, the weever fish would. Scarborough is famous for them. They lurk half-hidden in the sand below shallow water, stinging spines at the ready, and when groups of unsuspecting children run into their midst they are all stung together. To the Casualty staff the sign that weever fish have hit the beaches is a crowd of youngsters limping out of a single ambulance. The nurses thought the treatment had been the subject of debate in the medical press, though I had to confess I had missed it. The disagreement had been between steroids and calamine lotion, but the Scarborough solution was neither of these. Here they plunge an affected foot into a pail of hot water in which the weever fish toxin degenerates. I imagined the extraordinary scene – ranks of children, each with a therapeutic bucket – and secretly hoped it might happen while I was there.

Bank holidays meant trouble to Casualty staff as they brought together a dangerous combination of sun and liquor, both quick to go to the heads of the youths, mainly though not exclusively the men, arriving in the town in bus loads. Scarborough Hospital had watched it happen often and had patched up the results. Stag night brawls, raised voices outside pubs, clashes between trippers from Middlesbrough and Bradford, they all led to Casualty sooner or later. One of the nurses, John Henderson, had seen a teenager with a broken arm from being thrown in the harbour, another whose adversary had bitten off his nose. He blamed the climate. 'If it's a warm, balmy night,' said John, 'people will kick the shit out of each other.'

Sometimes the street fights continued in hospital, as the opponents queued impatiently side by side to present their injuries. Or else someone fresh from one battle would reach hospital looking for more of the same and needing only eye contact as provocation. Even for the staff casualty can be a frightening place and some departments around the country have taken to employing security guards to protect them.

Saturday in mid-season, the Scarborough nurses agreed, was not a time they relished. On a bad night, of which there were many, the waiting room quickly filled with arguments and abuse, punches were thrown and many patients were careless about where they emptied their stomachs and bladders. It could be an ugly, chaotic scene but the staff talked about it with the same sanguine shrug that they applied to all the failings and foibles of their clientele. There are some occupations, Casualty nurse being one, that, by making the average person shudder, help those who work in them to carry on. As long as everyone else gasped at how awful their job was, they could keep going.

Many of the summer season injuries, however, were self-inflicted, though accidentally. There was always someone with diabetes who overdid the cream-cakes, always someone who lodged a fish bone in his throat. And at least one crowd of teenagers every year would like the look of a crop of mushrooms in a field, not realizing until it was too late that what they were feasting on was a hallucinogenic fungus.

Then there was the sun, capable of catching holiday-makers unawares, over-heating the elderly and burning the young. 'It happens at the same time every year,' said John. 'The first week of sunshine and everyone flings their clothes off. Our place is full of people needing treatment for burns. Particularly the Scots, they're too sensitive. The old folk have the opposite problem. They keep everything on and they bake. It's a busy week for us. Even the dogs in the town are affected by the heat. It makes them bite.'

The new moon too was looked on as a bad omen; the nurses insisted that a fresh lunar cycle could herald the arrival in Casualty of a wave of self-destructive overdoses. It is amazing how many hospital staff, especially those who work through the night, believe in the power of the full moon, how often they will tell you tales of true 'lunatics', turned like a tide or a werewolf from one state to another by its evolution. It may be an example of how tenaciously medicine clings to the hocus-pocus to which it was once closely bound. Or it may arise from a love of superstition among those who practise medicine, a whimsical reaction to the current supremacy of science in the subject. Or, I suppose, it may be true.

Ten-thirty on Sunday mornings was equally, if more prosaically, a busy time, being the hour of the churchgoers, striding out too fast and collapsing with exhaustion when it was warm or aggravating their angina if there was a facing wind. 'It's a hilly town,' Chris Hughes explained, 'and some older visitors find the walk up to church too much for them.' You could set your watch by the sort of people who came through the Casualty door.

Chris, John and the others could have plied me all day with recollections; and what they were describing, the treatment of so many illnesses in a holiday town, was something more than medicine. It was a desperate defensive action, a battle against an ingenious foe capable of altering its appearance with infinite variety. The enemy was the fragility of the public, its tendency to come to grief in the pursuit of pleasure; it thrived on recklessness and complacency and dreamed up something new for every season. No holiday activity was too innocent to end on a stretcher, no promenader was ever completely safe.

The nurses who picked up the pieces could list the medical hazard affecting any vacation, from the parachutists with their awkward landings to the dehydrated trekkers brought in off the North Yorkshire Moors. Even less arduous endeavours, like country and western dancing at one of the local holiday camps for which Scarborough is famous, were risky. If someone at the hoedown didn't crush an ankle against the dance floor, the singer would break one by leaping off the stage. Chris and John remembered a Territorial Army weekend when no fewer than 250 cadets simultaneously went down with a stomach bug, as if responding *en masse* to a military order. And they could still picture the camper who turned up clutching the snake that had bitten him, an image that would cross my mind again later in the day.

The more we talked about how busy and unpredictable their job could be, the more it emphasized how quiet the department had appeared ever since my arrival. The cubicles remained empty and the waiting area free of snakes and sunburn. Even the jellyfish around the shore seemed to have taken a day off. I left the nurses where I had met them, in their staff room resting and reading but fully aware, like anyone in the emergency services, that the torpor which had descended on their workplace could at any moment be replaced by the most hectic and harrowing crisis. The one thing they could not predict was what it would look like this time.

I made my way to the hub of Scarborough's accommodation industry, the collection of hotels and boarding-houses just inland from the South Bay, noting the 'No Vacancies' signs that seemed to have been placed in every window. When you are looking for somewhere to stay, no expression is quite as smug as 'No Vacancies' but to the hoteliers and landlords it is probably written with relief that the late summer bank holiday has not let them down.

But if the desertion felt by many holiday towns, always attributed to the allure of the Costa del Sol, was less evident in Scarborough, who were the people who still came here, who were filling all the hotels? The boisterous day-trippers described by the nurses at the local hospital were nowhere to be seen. In fact the streets in this part of the town were quiet and only once in a while did a couple, usually around pensionable age, appear heading for the Esplanade above the beach, walking with that exaggerated slowness that is often used in taking the sea air. Through the windows I could see guests in their identical lounges, lit through low-level lampshades. Full hotels and empty streets: it seemed to me an image of decline, despite the 2 million visitors.

But for some it served its purpose, a point that became clear as I reached the head of the cliff where several of those who had ventured out to face the breeze were wheelchair-bound. To them it must have appeared a pleasant, spacious resort, its wide outlook round the bay and out over the North Sea a brief antidote to the limitations of immobility. And, up here at least, the atmosphere was peaceful even though the wind off the sea was accelerating. From where I stood, it was easy to see holidays as the pursuit of health, which in Scarborough is how they also began.

Before Elizabeth Farrow came across the spring that turned Scarborough into a spa town, its most noteworthy visitors were the Vikings and other northern warriors who burned it down or built it up according to their needs and, later, the tradesmen and mediaeval novelty acts who constituted Scarborough Fair – and who included bogus medical men selling quack remedies. Mrs Farrow was the wife of a well-off bailiff who himself was concerned enough about the health of his burgh to found a charity hospital. But her serendipitous finding in 1626 – she is supposed to have spotted the spring because of the discoloration it caused in the rocks near the shore – was of benefit to a different class of local society. With her encouragement the water was soon being swallowed in drawing-rooms throughout Scarborough and within a few years it was attracting the nobility from all over Yorkshire, who applied its healing properties to whatever they believed was wrong with their constitution. Throughout the century it was a regular summer haunt for health-seeking gentry. When Daniel Defoe passed through in the 1720s, he referred to 'a great deal of good company here drinking the waters, who came not only from all the north of England, but even from Scotland'.

Defoe liked Scarborough and refused to mock its activities, as he had done in Bath. His comments on the spa water itself – it was said to be unusually bitter – were confined to a chemical analysis. 'It is hard to describe the taste of the waters,' he wrote; 'they are apparently tinged with a collection of mineral salts, as of vitriol, alum, iron, and perhaps sulphur, and taste evidently of alum.'

By the end of the seventeenth century the town authorities had constructed a cistern to collect Mrs Farrow's discovery and had tried to block the approach of the tide to prevent the unique flavour of the spa from being contaminated by brine. But this unwelcoming attitude to the North Sea was soon dropped as a concurrence of changing social and medical opinion turned Scarborough into one of the country's most fashionable destinations, a transformation owing much to the new-found popularity of sea water.

At first the value of the sea was medicinal, a logical extension of the universal belief that immersion and ingestion of waters, particularly the unpalatable kind, were good for you. Doctors promoted this notion, directing their patients to the coast to inhale the bracing sea breeze, something that from the evidence of my visit Scarborough was well able to provide. From this supposed cure it was only a short step to sea bathing and then sea drinking. In 1752 Richard Russell, a doctor living in Brighton – another town that was benefiting from the idea – wrote 'A Dissertation on the use of Sea Water', in which he observed its palliative effects on the multifarious diseases of urban life. The sea, it seemed, could remedy anything and the leisured classes swarmed to the coast to collect their dose.

There seems little doubt that the prescription worked. Scarborough and its southern rivals would not have flourished unless they had been genuinely capable of invigorating their sickly visitors. But the active ingredient in their success, unless modern medicine has got it wrong, could only have been the opportunities they offered to lift the spirits and relax the limbs, to gaze at their panoramic outlook, to rest, stroll and ponder.

For a time Scarborough, with its medicinal spring and its seaside location, was able to boast a combination of attractions that no other resort or spa town could match. But another shift in social preference led people to come here simply for enjoyment. Previously towns at the coast had been looked on as wild, storm-battered places but the experiences of those who convalesced by the sea altered this impression. Walking, swimming and admiring the view grew to be valued in themselves rather than as part of a medical treatment. In Scarborough the spa became less important than the sea and the solace the town offered to the exhausted rich was no longer alone in drawing the crowds. Now a new interloper, the holiday-maker, appeared in search of pleasure. When in 1789 George III waded into the sea at Melcombe, the fun of seaside bathing was officially endorsed and thriving resorts soon dotted the country's coastline. But in the North the wealthiest and most popular was Scarborough. By the start of the nineteenth century almost one house in ten was renting out its rooms and, I imagined, the first 'No Vacancies' signs were being written.

The initial spa buildings were constructed over 200 years ago but the cliff tramcars by which I descended to the sea front did not begin transporting people between the spa and the residences high above the South Bay until 1875. I wandered along to where the modern buildings stand but, as there seemed to be no one there, I did not stay long. Peering in at the concert arena, I could see rows of unoccupied chairs, not unlike the scene I had left behind in Casualty, facing an empty stage. In one corner of the hall there was an audience of two, waiting and chewing.

Down at the beach the picture was the same: a handful of determined bathers and not much more. Where was everyone? Further along the bay, beside stacks of unemployed deck-chairs, I could see figures moving and I set off in their direction along the shoreline.

Daniel Defoe would have been shocked at the appearance of the sea. 'Here,' he wrote, 'is such a plenty of all sorts of fish, that I have hardly seen the like, and, in particular, here we saw turbets of three quarters of a hundred weight, and yet their flesh eat exceedingly fine when taken new.' Today he would go hungry. Like most of Britain's coastal resorts (it is certainly not the worst), Scarborough has a hygiene problem. The North Sea has had its fill of effluent waste and has begun throwing it back at the beaches in waves opaque with filth and micro-organisms. Times have changed: no one now would drink sea water for the sake of their health.

The water that day was thick with seaweed but even so a layer of scum was clearly visible over its surface, and when it reached the beach it turned into a dirty froth that stained the sand. The local authorities, I was told during my trip, were concerned about the contamination and planned to reverse it but the only positive remark I heard about the current condition of South Bay was that North Bay was much worse.

Although their numbers were still thin, I had by now finally come across some holiday-makers and there was no doubt that they were enjoying themselves despite the strengthening wind and the state of the sea. One young boy was paddling in his anorak, another was pacing backwards and forwards in front of the waves as if on guard duty against the microbes. In the same repetitive way garlanded donkeys were plodding up and down with tiny infants riding them, screaming hilariously. Here and there families were using the wet sand as a cricket pitch. The whole scene could have been transplanted into the 1950s and no one would have spotted anything out of place.

As the arrival of railways in the nineteenth century made Scarborough more accessible, its amenities began to spill inland from around the bays, its population multiplied and elegant hotels sprang up on every newly built street. But the greatest change was that the town ceased to be a haven for the monied classes. By the 1870s barbers' apprentices and bootblacks on day trips from Leeds were spoiling the peace of their betters with their rowdiness and their love of ale.

Although residents may have resented the intrusion, there was no holding back social progress. Scarborough in season was soon awash with pedlars and freak shows, some of which had not been seen there since the mediaeval fair but which now returned to cater for the invasion of working men and their families. Donkeys were ridden along the sands for the first time and 'what the butler saw' slot machines offered a novel titillation. The medical con men also came back, selling worthless panaceas and reading the bumps in their customers' skulls. For those who preferred a more traditional placebo, spa water minerals were on sale as 'Scarborough salts'. Holidays and the resorts where they happened were no longer reserved for the rich, although the social classes kept their distance from each other for many more years, aided in Scarborough's case by the presence of two separate bays.

Sitting well back from the water, near steps up to the road, there was a family group sheltering behind a wind-break which fell over every few minutes. They might have been posing for a snapshot by Cartier-Bresson; they sat together facing different directions, the mother fleshy and in sunglasses, a girl feeding a baby, her brothers drawing in the sand or staring into space beside a man in the only deck-chair. But what made this family unusual was that they seemed to be the subject of a news report or even a television documentary because a film crew was hovering round them trying to find the best angle to shoot from. The men with the cameras wore T-shirts printed with the name of a beach in Florida and from the quizzical expressions on their faces they seemed to think they were filming a separate species.

Their activities were watched with distant interest by passers-by in the increasingly busy street above the sand. There were women pushing prams, elderly couples buried under caps and scarves, and on one bench what appeared to be three generations of males, eating ice-creams in unison. Across the road stood the Futurist theatre, in fact a relic of the past; there was ten-pin bowling and a variety show that promised 'all laughter'. A topless tourist bus labelled 'Appleby's Seaside Spectacular' chugged past, its sparse passengers heavily dressed against the cold.

There was something admirable about the town front – how it had stuck to its Englishness and how resolutely its visitors set about making the most of it – but in the way that going down with your ship is admirable. Promoting an old-fashioned charm is an unsafe strategy because it relies on holiday-makers to maintain a constant preference, something that is not a part of the holiday ethos, at least not any more. The modern vacation is a throw-away activity, fed by the lure of new experience, and just as the cures which first brought crowds to Scarborough are no longer considered effective, the novelties that placed it among the most successful of resorts cannot go on for ever being thought of as fun.

It was a dangerous spot where I had been walking, I was told by the ambulancemen with whom I spent most of the remaining daylight hours. They did not mean the South Bay, where they were rarely called, except to something unusual like an oil spill from an offshore tanker (though it wasn't clear what was expected of them in such cases) but the broad marine road which looped round the castle remains to reach North Bay. This was an exposed route and the wind off the sea had seemed stronger than ever. I had taken a perfunctory glance at North Bay, assured myself that nothing much was going on and retreated back through the town where there was more bustle and less weather. What I had arranged next was a rendezvous with another of Scarborough's front-line medical services.

The ambulance station had the look of a warehouse and the air of a waiting-room. There were two crews and so far no calls, but Geoff and the others gave the impression that passing the time was a skill they had acquired early. The road between the bays, they told me, was notorious because on a stormy day the waves could surge over the railings and on to the pavement, dragging pedestrians back into the sea where the chance of survival was zero. The Scarborough ambulance-men had known people to drown that way but they also remembered cases where victims had leapt clear only to land in the path of a passing car. For drivers too it was a perilous highway with a sudden switch of direction at its north end; once in a while someone misjudged his speed and ploughed into the railings. It was a type of emergency they had all been called to at some time.

Attending road accidents was a frequent part of their work through-out the year – the holiday season did not so much alter what ambu-lances did as multiply it – but most were located not in the centre of the town but on the outskirts and approach roads. 'Every day we see at least two or three RTAs,' said Geoff, using the abbreviation for road traffic accident that is part of the Casualty lingo. 'This week we've had two that were fatal. The problem is the holiday-makers, particularly the day-trippers who come by car. There are more of them now because there's less money around and people have to settle for short visits. They get frustrated when they get caught in traffic on the way here, so they overtake when they shouldn't.'

Geoff and his colleagues knew a lot about death on the road and one of the things they knew best was how illogical it was. They had seen drivers step unharmed out of crushed vehicles, and even react impatiently when asked about their well-being, and they had found others dead at the wheels of cars with hardly a dent. And like everyone else who routinely faces horror in their work they had learned to talk about it dispassionately.

I was there to join them on duty when the next call came in but, just as in casualty earlier, the requests for help had dried up. There was nothing to do except wait while the ambulancemen filled me in on the details of their job. The farms in the area could be as lethal as the roads, they said, and they had seen farm workers lose limbs in the machinery used in baling. At least these were cases that they felt able to help; the worst times were when they were summoned to a cardiac arrest and gave heart massage for half an hour on the journey to hospital, only for the patient to be pronounced dead on arrival; futility was exhausting. Overall it was varied work: insecure scaffolding, ugly domestic rows, collapse on the moors – someone always dialled for an ambulance. They were high on profile but, they added with a hint of envy directed at firemen, low on glamour.

Bank holiday Saturday could be a day of mayhem and they were expecting a deluge of calls despite the dearth so far. Somewhere in Scarborough a drunk man would be preparing to collide with a pavement. Or walk on glass in bare feet. Or pick a fight. Stick around, they said, the action wouldn't be long.

I looked out of the window to see that the weather had turned mild, drank more coffee, and ran out of questions. A few more minutes, I thought, and then I would have to leave and go looking for a hotel. But a moment later the emergency phone rang. One crew ran for its waiting vehicle and I ran after them but somehow they had mistaken what I was there for and they drove off before I reached them. Having waited for hours for that first call, I had missed it.

The next one came in seconds later: woman found unconscious at home, no other details. I jumped in the back beside the oxygen supply and the defibrillator, the electrical instrument used to re-start the heart, which rattled and bounced as we pulled out of the station and set off the siren. Children waved from the roadside and cars moved slowly aside to let us through. The holiday traffic turned it into a laborious journey but the distance was short and we were soon being flagged down by our patient's neighbour, who told us it was she who had raised the alarm.

We followed her direction up a narrow stair to a flat, carrying everything for a resuscitation. But it wasn't needed: the woman was motionless on the floor but able to speak. She had taken some sleeping pills, she said. The neighbour whispered that she had been depressed, that she had become a recluse since the death of her husband a few months earlier. On the journey from the street to Scarborough Hospital there was no need for a siren. The woman sat in the back of the ambulance in silence, wrapped in a blanket. It might have been a holiday town at the height of its season but this kind of emergency was routine all over the country.

When we reached the Casualty department I said hello to the nurses I had met several hours before. Activity in the waiting-area was stepping into a higher gear. The neat rows of seats were thrown out of line, curtains were being drawn around cubicles, the place was steadily filling and restless patients were asking how much longer they would have to stay there. We delivered our woman and returned quickly to the early evening air, now completely calm. It seemed that the town and its hospital was after all heading for a balmy night.

But there was still the matter of where I would sleep. I had already tried countless hotels in the town centre and around the Esplanade without success. Now I asked at a few more, but with no better result. I drove north to the nearby village of Scalby, the first parish of William Mompesson, key figure in the Eyam plague, whose story was the subject of my next journey, but everywhere there too was full. It was late. I turned west, travelling inland on the Pickering road, stopping at every pub that claimed to rent out rooms. All taken, they each told me, with more pride than sympathy.

I had lost the holiday spirit but at least I had come prepared. I had a tent in the back of the car and a few miles outside Scarborough I turned off the main road towards a campsite. It was in darkness and looked full but I sneaked in and put up my canvas on a grass verge, scrambling on the ground and recalling momentarily the snake story I had heard in Casualty. In the morning I found the proprietor and asked the price of a night but when he saw me he too lost the holiday spirit. It seemed I had committed the most wicked of crimes: I had slept in a place with no vacancies. I had broken the rules of the resort, he fumed, and I was evicted before breakfast.

TEN

The Derbyshire Peak

I ENTERED Derbyshire where the Pennines peter out, crossing the combination of hills and moorland around Buxton, 'so inhospitable, so rugged and so wild a place,' according to Daniel Defoe, that 'the gentry choose to reside at Derby rather than upon their estates'. Now it is an area that people flock to, one of those places where, if you stand in it for long enough, every hill walker in Britain will nod to you.

Derbyshire is England compressed into one county. There are industrial towns and well-heeled villages, highways blocked by tractors and hilltop passes blocked, from time to time, by snow. In the north there are grey peaks, in the south there are brooks that really do babble. It has its own cakes and its own ale. There are moments when, travelling through it, you feel in danger of breaking into a morris dance.

But one characteristic of the landscape sets it aside from most of the country: the limestone cliffs that line the roadside and loom in the distance. Where the surface of the hills is broken, layers of off-white rock stand out, looking ready to crumble; these are the edges of underground strata that are the dominating element of the region's geology, as well as the root of its diseases.

Not that the Derbyshire Peaks are all chalk, and neither have all the illnesses there been a direct product of the limestone itself; the health of the population has owed as much to what lies within these craggy layers as to what they themselves are made of. Where I was now driving is famous for mining lead, so much so that the excavations are part of a well-trodden tourist circuit, and to the east lies the county's coalfields: two industries with their own pattern of disease. And shortly before I arrived in the district, high concentrations of radon gas had been found in Buxton and neighbouring towns. Radon has increasingly been blamed as a cause of malignancy, second only to smoking in the case of lung cancer (though a long way behind), and its contamination of the Derbyshire air follows seepage from the decaying uranium deep within the limestone strata, an echo of Sellafield.

I heard during my visit that lime was, inevitably I suppose, one of the major ingredients in the medicinal waters that seem to abound in the Peaks, such as those at Buxton. Defoe, although he looked on the appearance of the spring there as distinctly ordinary, thought they were capable of 'wonderful cures' and of such a perfect temperature that 'you . . . can hardly be persuaded to come out of the bath when you are in'.

Lime in the local water also seems to have been the cause of 'Derbyshire neck', the colloquial name for the goitre that used to be endemic here. In 1802 Thomas Beddoes reported a widespread belief that the water of melted snow was the cause of Derbyshire neck. Certainly the occurrence of identical thyroid swelling in the Alps, where it was first decribed, would support that view. But if melted snow was part of the problem, it was through contributing to a diet low in iodine.

The thyroid gland, which lies at the front of the neck straddling the larynx, takes up iodine from the circulation and uses it to construct hormones that regulate the rate of the body's metabolism. Too little available iodine causes the thyroid to enlarge in an attempt to compensate for its underactivity, the swollen gland being known as a goitre. But if the iodine shortage is too great, the thyroid cannot keep the body's chemical activities going and the resulting symptoms are low temperature, a slow heart, weight gain, hair loss, a husky voice, general sluggishness and eventually mental failure leading to dementia. When babies are affected congenitally, their appearance is striking. Their abdomens are distended, their skin and hair are dry and their tongues are large and protruding. They seem listless and feed badly. If untreated they are damaged intellectually, hence the the modern slang meaning attached to the medical name for their condition, cretinism.

Goitre, thyroid failure and cretinism occur together in parts of the world where the dietary intake of iodine is low. These are areas where the local water has little iodine in it, far from the coast and its iodine-rich seafoods, usually mountainous regions such as the Himalayas and the Andes. Medical reports during the nineteenth century, before more balanced diets and iodine supplementation, suggested that these conditions were not uncommon, and in Britain they were probably widespread. But it was Derbyshire that achieved the distinction of being associated with them, of attaching its name to its own medical disorder and the reason probably lay in the limestone. If Derbyshire neck was genuinely more common in Derbyshire, it may have been because the calcium in the local lime-rich water became bound to the iodine dissolved there, thus removing it from solution before it could reach the county's water supply.

In a sense Derbyshire neck was the reason I was travelling. It summed up the point of the whole journey and explained why I was now stuck in a queue of caravans. It was a medical condition that not only revealed something fundamental about the character of the place where it arose, it also spelled out its origin in its name; few diseases did that. There were many syndromes with the names of famous doctors attached to them but what did they reveal about the culture or structure of the country that produced them? Here was what I had been looking for, a disorder that hinted at its local geology. But here also, I had to admit, was a medical problem that people no longer developed. I had set out a hundred years too late to find Derbyshire neck.

When the convoy that had escorted me for ten miles or more finally reached Matlock Bath, I slipped out and parked beside the River Derwent near a ragged rock face called the Heights of Abraham. The Peak District Mining Museum, a celebration of Derbyshire's lead industry, was easy to find if difficult to reach by road. Fortunately Len Willies, the founder of the museum to whom I had spoken a few days earlier, had hung around despite my lateness. Len, who described himself as a 'historian, geologist and archaeologist', had a historian's habit of talking in the present tense about events that took place centuries ago, as if they were too vivid to be left in the past.

Derbyshire was once, three hundred years ago, the hub of lead production in Europe. And in the north of the county, around Stoney Middleton, both smelting and underground mining still take place, though there is little connection between them as most of the ore brought out of the mine is exported. At least as early as Roman times lead from the area was being transported overseas, a fact confirmed a few years ago when the wreck of a Roman ship discovered off the coast of Brittany – Len was cagey about precisely where the wreck lay – was found to contain lead ingots from the region. The Romans needed lead to construct something central to their idea of civilization, their baths and pipes, and the English from the Middle Ages onwards used it in one of their own preoccupations, church roofs. Nowadays it goes into batteries.

Surface mining too still continues near Bradwell but, Len told me, the presence of lead in Derbyshire is not confined to the many seams. Traces are found in soil and even in house-dust in many parts of the county and can enter the roots of plants including those that are eaten by animals, although its penetration of the food chain is said to be slight. Nevertheless, there are occasional cases of lead poisoning among animals such as horses and cows resulting from ingestion of contaminated grass roots. Other animals are even more at risk. Len told me that one way of pinpointing ancient lead workings is to ask if anyone in an area keeps chickens. On lead-rich ground it is impossible to do so as the birds' penchant for eating grit means they are soon poisoned.

And humans, I wondered? The tiny amounts of lead that do enter the population do not come from eating contaminated vegetables but from licking fingers that have touched dusty leaves. Another source of polluted dust used to be the clothing of people who worked in the smelting industry, who unknowingly carried the lead home where their children, more susceptible to its effects, could ingest it. As recently as fifteen or twenty years ago, said Len, the nail-biting offspring of smelters could accumulate significant quantities in their circulation. Yet cases of poisoning were rare then and are even rarer now, since the industry stepped up its measures to remove and monitor lead levels in its employees through a combination of sprays and medical checks. The local water too is surprisingly free of lead salts, which appear to dissolve only slightly in lime-rich streams and reservoirs. In fact, although in some of Britain's cities old lead water pipes are regarded with suspicion and have been blamed for aggression and low intelligence, in Derbyshire the old lead mine soughs – horizontal tunnels originally dug as drains for the mines – act here and there as part of the water supply system.

However infrequent lead poisoning may be nowadays, it is a medical condition as old as Hippocrates, quite literally, because it was he who in 370 BC first attributed an attack of abdominal colic to lead. His patient was employed as an extractor of metal from ore. Saturnism – named after Saturn, the alchemists' name for lead – was thus among the earliest of occupational diseases, and this was not the last time that it was to break new ground in industrial medicine because over 2,000 years later in Britain it was the first occupational disorder to be a specific target of legislation.

Between these two events came Derbyshire's rise to fame as the supplier of lead to most of the known world. Once the Romans had left, Len explained, the trade went through a lull as few lead-containing roofs were constructed, and the lead that became available through the pillaging of towns was enough to satisfy demand. In the thirteenth century the industry picked up after metallic lead was used to fill in crevices in the rock foundations of the Tower of London's new buildings, and after white lead, a pigment composed of hydroxide and carbonate salts, was used in the painting of Edward I's bed-chamber. But there were major setbacks to come. First of these was the Black Death, which wiped out so many people that every trade in the land went into decline. Then there was the Reformation, when monasteries were torn down and the lead from their roofs recycled, undermining the whole European market.

But around 1600, thanks to better methods of excavation, Derbyshire lead rose to prominence and poisoned workmen became, if not commonplace, then unsurprising. The manifestations of lead toxicity are numerous: colic, blindness, fits, anaemia and kidney failure are all possible effects. Particularly vulnerable is the nerve supply to the limbs, resulting in wrist and foot drop but Len did not believe that foot drop had been common in the mines. Even though the miners wore a special sort of clog which can still be found at the bottom of the main shafts, this was more to protect against the damp conditions underground than to compensate for nerve damage. Yet the most famous effect of lead intoxication, at least in medical circles, is also the most innocuous: a blue line on the gums (some say it is black) from the deposition of lead sulphide, the same mineral that was and still is extracted in a crystalline form called galena from Derbyshire rocks. The blue line of lead poisoning is one of those medical signs that most modern doctors know about but hardly any have seen. Yet in Derbyshire it was well known and may have been made more common there by the county's interest in farming, or rather in eating its own farm produce. The sulphur in eggs was supposed to react with lead in the circulation to produce the blue line. So if your chickens hadn't already died of it themselves, their eggs might warn you of the danger of lead in the locality.

As Len was keen to point out, the risks in lead mining were as much in the mining as they were in the lead. To get to the veins of galena, which could be anything from thirty metres to a few centimetres wide, a series of tunnels had to be burrowed through the Derbyshire rock. Many of them were cramped and wet, and some of them liable to cave in, especially when gunpowder replaced the pickaxe as the main means of excavation in the late eighteenth century. Limestone slabs threatened to fall from the stratified tunnel walls and, as in the coal-mines, gases leaked out of the fractured seams, in particular carbon dioxide, which escaped from the abundant layers of shale.

Where the miners worked was damp and suffocating enough to be blamed for the poor chests and painful joints from which many of them suffered, and the chief safety precaution of the time, a lighted candle, was adopted with this in mind, as it would not burn where there was insufficient oxygen. But according to Len the mine managers made sure the candle was held some distance from the vein where the men were working, so that it was able to keep burning while they choked.

Several decades after the supremacy of Derbyshire lead had faded, a doctor called William Webb wrote in the *British Medical Journal* about the health of miners in the county. It was a noticeably positive report. Despite their 'many hardships and numerous privations' he believed they rarely died before they were sixty. Occupational injuries did not appear to occur with the frequency seen in the coal-fields during the same period – the 1850s – and gas explosions were rare as were fatal accidents which, Dr Webb stated, 'happen mostly to old miners who have grown careless'. But by the time of his observations, said Len, there were few people working in the mines and what he found could not be taken as typical of the industry at its earlier peak.

Nevertheless Webb did draw attention to what he called the 'general prostration of the system' which in his view resulted from breathing too little oxygen and too much carbon dioxide underground. Even the healthy miner could 'generally be pointed out by his pallid face' but many suffered from breathlessness, headache and a slow, feeble pulse. To be cured miners had to rest and eat a decent diet, Webb opined, but it was equally important that they should take preventive action at work by carrying not a candle but a supply of quicklime, calcium hydroxide, capable of removing carbon dioxide from the atmosphere.

The sickly complexion of the Derbyshire miner was something on which Defoe had also remarked nearly a hundred years earlier when, as he crossed Brassington Moor, a few miles south of Matlock, a man suddenly emerged in front of him from a crack in the hillside. 'He was as lean as a skeleton,' wrote Defoe, 'pale as a dead corpse, his hair and beard a deep black, his flesh lank, and, as we thought, something of the colour of lead itself.' Defoe thought the miner looked as if he had risen from 'the dark regions', a hell in the heart of England, and he reacted as any Englishman would; he bought the man a drink.

Yet it was not the miners but the smelters who ran the highest risk of illness from contact with lead. While underground workers had to ingest it before they were intoxicated, smelters manning the furnaces could also inhale it throughout their working day. By the nineteenth century, although the mining itself was in decline, smelting was still advancing and the furnaces at this time were notoriously poisonous, being equipped with bellows that blew fumes straight at the men who stoked them. Meanwhile the dust in the foundries settled on clothes and skin and easily reached the mouth. The only 'protection' from illness was for many years a high fat diet, which was believed to reduce the absorption of lead from the gut. Then in the 1880s a new prophylactic was given to smelters: a sulphuric acid drink made more palatable by the addition of sugar and lemon. The sulphate in the acid was known to react with the lead carbonate of white lead to form lead sulphate, thought to be insoluble. But as Len related, it was not until forty years later that someone tested the theory. As it turned out, the absorption of lead in its sulphate form was even greater.

But a more important measure was also taken in the late nineteenth century. In 1883 the Factories (Prevention of Lead Poisoning) Act became the first industrial law directed at a specific medical condition. Ventilation was improved and factories were obliged to provide separate meal rooms. From that moment cases of lead poisoning were seen to dwindle. But then so did the industry.

Smelting continues in Derbyshire but galena is only one of the ores to go into the furnaces. From fluorspar, the 'flowing rock', comes fluoride for toothpaste; barium is extracted from baryte and what is not used to drill through mud under the North Sea is converted to barium meals to explore our stomachs. It is a small industry now but it has retained the reputation for safety that the 1883 Act established. Yet even then smelting was past its prime; economic boom and the protection of life and limb seem always to be separate phases of industrial development, never simultaneous.

I left Len Willies and joined the procession of traffic heading north, stopping in Lathkill Dale to look at the old mine workings, the remains of an aqueduct and some aborted tunnels a few metres long. If Derbyshire is England in miniature and lead mining an English occupation (begun by the Romans, remarked on by Defoe – you can't get more English than that), then the diseases it caused, as well as the legal protection that followed, must be essentially English too, products of a partnership between natural resources and human adversity. In William Webb's article in the *British Medical Journal* he offered the opinion that the Derbyshire lead miner was healthier than might be expected because of three possessions: a pleasant cottage, a supportive wife and his own cow. As a portrait of the nation down the centuries, it would be hard to beat.

The village of Eyam in north Derbyshire lies in the valley of Hope, a location that might have pleased John Bunyan, given what happened here three centuries ago. At that time Eyam was surrounded by busy lead mines and it was the widow of a miner who played a central part in the story which the village celebrates every summer.

It is not a place of natural beauty, though on the day I turned up it had dolled itself up with moss, lentils, berries and hydrangea petals in the pagan craft of well-dressing. It was August bank holiday, a weekend when Eyam soaks up outsiders not just to admire its tradition of worshipping water but to join in a religious service that recalls the arrival of bubonic plague in the parish in 1665. Of course it is not known exactly when the plague reached Eyam, or exactly how, although the conventional account is so appealingly tragic that no one wants to disbelieve it.

A handful of people slogging up the hill towards the church were a sign that today's commemoration was hotting up and I followed them until they stopped beside a small terrace of houses, the plague cottages, where it all began. It was here that the lead miner's widow Mary Cooper lived with her sons Edward and Jonathan, and it was at this time of year that she is thought to have taken in a temporary lodger, George Viccars, an itinerant tailor. At the beginning of September Viccars became feverish and by the sixth or seventh of the month he had died.

The death of a travelling salesman in itself would have caused little stir in the village but within ten days there was a cluster of cases of similar fever in and around the Cooper home. Edward Cooper died on 22 September and before the end of the month there had been two deaths in the Thorpe family who lived on one side of the Coopers, one in the Hawksworth family who lived on the other side, and a further death in the Sydall household across the street. It must have been quickly apparent that plague had struck and, judging by how soon the better-off were able to leave Eyam, panic was the one thing that spread more rapidly than the bacillus. And with good reason, 1665 being the year of London's notorious Great Plague.

It must also have been at this early stage that suspicions about the source of the disease were first directed towards the chest of clothes that had arrived from London for George Viccars a few days before he died, although it was another fifty years before this version of events was first written down. The bacterium that causes plague, *Yersinia pestis*, lives on the fleas found on the black rat and at times other mammals. So, even if Viccars's complaints about flea-bites as recorded in some narratives are late embellishments, the belief among the survivors of Eyam that the plague reached them in his clothes box is not impossible.

Yet credibility is not what makes legends last and I wondered as the village prepared for its ceremony whether the story of the Eyam plague had been kept alive so long by the disturbing element of chance that it entails. Chance, and the uncertainty that is inevitably part of it, is unsettling and cannot easily be tolerated. Superstitions and religions have been developed to make sense of what otherwise seem like chance events. Science itself, which at first sight looks to be in opposition to religion, carries the same purpose: to give predictability to occurrences that might otherwise appear random. We go to great lengths to avoid the conclusion that things happen by chance, we look for a pattern or a culprit, because if there is neither of these our sense of security is undermined. So any tragedy that afflicts a person or place for no particular reason is especially threatening. Just as the Black Death could have arrived at any port in England, the garments George Viccars received from plague-ridden London could have reached him at many points along his route around the country. There is no obvious reason why Eyam should have been the place but as events turned out that was where he grew ill and where a chain of disastrous and noble events was begun in the lives of the villagers. Whether it is true or not, the story of the infested clothes box is one of the reasons that what happened in Eyam has remained so compelling.

It was approaching the time for the annual procession to Cucklet Delph and I wanted to look around the Church of St Lawrence before it was under way. The church was enjoying its most popular day of the year and was entertaining its visitors with a billboard display explaining how the plague had struck, an account that was both shocking and heroic. The Eyam story as presented by the church frieze was the authorized version and there was also a series of stained glass windows depicting the arrival of the diseased cloth, the demise of Viccars and the camaraderie of William Mompesson and Thomas Stanley, the men whose selfless courage added to the poignancy of the outbreak. Yet the human characteristics essential to what took place in Eyam were more mundane than heroism and in a way more interesting; they were ignorance, superstition and guilt.

In the seventeenth century the idea that microscopic life forms were responsible for the plague would have seemed fanciful. Instead the cures and palliatives, a reflection of the medicine of the day, relied on herbs and old wives' tales whose nature seemed to depend simply on whatever happened to grow locally. Aromatic plants such as feverfew and wormwood were supposed to abolish the fever while buboes, the unsightly swellings that gave the disease its name, were treated by drawing their infected contents to the surface where they could be released. To achieve this end, as the church display detailed, it was conventional to place the rump of a live chicken or a plucked pigeon over the plague sore until it had soaked up so much poison that the creature died. This sorry business was repeated until a bird survived or the patient perished, whichever came first.

Obviously such remedies were useless but some of them became part of a plague folklore which has not yet disappeared. So suddenly did the disease attack a community, so quickly did it wipe out its victims and their families, and so high was the mortality that its place in the hierarchy of human fears was guaranteed for centuries to come. Plague: the word still sounds malevolent and when used as a verb it implies something relentless. There have been no major outbreaks (and only a single minor one) in Britain since the one in Eyam but so completely had it infiltrated our thinking by then that its mark is still on the culture. There is the 'bless you' reflex when someone sneezes, one of the early symptoms. There is the 'ring o' roses' nursery rhyme, the rose being a nickname for the skin lesion that some cases developed as well as one of the flowers used to ward off infection, hence 'a pocketful of posies'. Atishoo, atishoo, we all fall down, and almost all those who contracted the disease did just that.

The terrible fear that plague aroused would have persuaded the villagers of Eyam to view their predicament as a punishment. Although the Church of St Lawrence offers a list of ludicrous cures, suggesting how primitive were the folk-beliefs surrounding the epidemic, it makes little of the moral response that must have followed. But a thin pamphlet on the outbreak written by John G. Clifford and sold in the church is less neglectful of the seventeenth-century religious view that such a pestilence was a judgement on the people who caught it.

The plague story is today made palatable only by the feeling that its danger is held at a safe distance, three centuries away. It all happened a long time ago and now we live in a more sophisticated age. The tales of therapeutic blossoms and chickens seem pathetic, misguided and primitive, a product of ignorance that progress and the passage of time have cleared away. But the moral explanation for illness that people believed in at the same time that they trusted in the healing power of the plucked pigeon has not gone, as the reaction to the spread of Aids in cities such as Edinburgh had shown.

Despite the many myths about what would spread or suppress the plague, it seems that only the falling temperature of late autumn kept the number of deaths down, the *Yersinia* bacterium being sensitive to cold. The register of victims, the pride of the church's exhibits, revealed this vividly. Five residents died in the parish in November, eight in December. In the first five months of 1666 a total of twenty villagers were killed by the illness. Although these figures meant that plague was still present, it must have seemed to some that the worst was over. There must also have been those who feared the return of warm weather in the summer.

Across the road from the church was a pub where I waited as the crowd that had gathered outside turned itself into a procession. A big man with a beard like a hedge was standing solidly in the middle of the street with a hymn book open at the ready. Suddenly the congregation was moving. I couldn't see the front of the cavalcade where I assumed the vicar of St Lawrence was stepping out ahead, but all attention at the back where I walked was focused on the bearded man who had burst into song like an explosion.

In June 1666 the fears of the Eyam survivors were realized and the young vicar William Mompesson made the decision for which the plague here is remembered. On the twelfth of the month there was an abrupt increase in the number of deaths, leading some later commentators to believe that the plague had switched to an even more lethal variant in which the main site of infection is the lungs. The total number of victims in June was twenty-one, the highest monthly figure since the previous October.

Mompesson was twenty-eight and had been in the parish with his wife Catherine and their two children for just over a year when the outbreak began, having come from Scalby, near Scarborough, in early 1664. In his work he was assisted by Thomas Stanley, a Puritan who had himself been rector until 1660, when the Royalist revival led clergymen of his persuasion to be deposed.

Throughout June the bodies mounted up too quickly for the local gravedigger to bury them and it was then that Mompesson and Stanley persuaded the villagers to take a decision of extraordinary self-sacrifice. To prevent the spread of the disease into neighbouring towns, no one else would leave Eyam. For the good of the whole region all villagers would remain close to the source of the infection. Most accounts of the plague accept the fact that Mompesson's children had been packed off to friends miles away before the quarantine was initiated but there is a less noble version that reverses this sequence of events. Either way, it seems likely that Mompesson wanted his whole family to escape but that Catherine insisted on staying to help him with his pastoral duties. Eyam was cut off from the rest of the county and had to rely on helpful – also relieved – outsiders who left food at designated points on the village boundary and who were paid with coins left in running water or vinegar, intended as disinfectant.

In July there were fifty-six deaths, in August seventy-eight, including Catherine Mompesson. By now some families had been almost destroyed. The Thorpe household, one of whom had been among the first victims, had lost six members. The Sydalls across the road had lost seven. One sixteen-day stretch had seen five of the Thornley family lose their lives. When the last death occurred on 1 November, the total stood at 259, out of a population calculated at the time to have been 350. This figure may have been a substantial underestimation, however, and probably omitted those who left the area as soon as the crisis emerged.

Both Mompesson and Stanley lived through the disaster, regularly holding religious services in a shallow valley a short walk from their church, known as Cucklet's Delph. Medical knowledge could not have been as rudimentary as the cock-eyed plague therapies now suggest because Mompesson had closed his church in case his congregation transmitted the disease to each other by standing close together inside the building. In fact the decision of the villagers to stay put for the sake of others shows that they were aware that the spread of infection was encouraged by contact or proximity.

I caught up with the front of the procession at Cucklet's Delph as the commemorative service of prayers and purpose-built Eyam hymns was beginning before a crowd of a few hundred residents, tourists and broadcasters. The theme was sacrifice. From where I was standing I could see the tower of the Church of St Lawrence through the trees that surround the Delph. By coincidence the end of August is the anniversary not only of the appearance of the plague but also of Catherine Mompesson's death and I had seen that by tradition someone had placed a ring of red roses on the monument to her in the churchyard.

The self-sacrifice in Eyam was heroic in a way but more than that it was pathetic and pitiful. I imagined Mompesson in August 1666 comforting one moribund person after another, seeing his wife and half his congregation fall fatally ill and somehow sticking to his decision that everyone should stay, even if it meant that everyone should die. Perhaps he managed it because of his faith, because of fear of making the situation worse or because the tragedy was so numbing that he could no longer see a way of altering the course of events. But how, I wondered, did he react when it was over? How did he begin again to plan what he did from one day to the next after a long period of being governed by something beyond his control? How did he find any interest in the minor worries of his parishioners or in the work of the church?

When the plague had finally left, Mompesson burned all his clothes and bed sheets and encouraged others to do the same. He remained in Eyam for four years, leaving in 1670, the year Thomas Stanley died, for a new post at Eakring in Lincolnshire. He remarried the same year. From then on biographical details are few but it appears that he lived quietly, submerging himself in the routine business of the clergy and turning down an offer of promotion. After what he had witnessed, he must have welcomed uneventful days and hoped that nothing of consequence would happen.

ELEVEN

East Anglia

ALGAE were in the news the day I arrived in East Anglia. Bulletins on my car radio announced with alarm the contamination of local reservoirs. Public officials warned the water could be fatally poisonous to pets. They were talking about blue-green algae but I had another species in mind: a seaweed called *Alcyonidium gelatinosum*, chief culprit in a condition bearing the glorious name of Dogger Bank itch, which I was beginning to fear did not exist.

For the moment the itch would have to wait. I had come to find out what I could about staying alive, something the residents of East Anglia did better than anyone else in the country. Mortality from heart disease was lower than in all other regions, and might be lower still if the many deaths from what used to be called old age were not conventionally recorded as cardiovascular in origin. In fact, if it were not for the sporadic rivalry of south-west England, East Anglia would have the lowest death rates from almost all major illnesses. It also admitted to the highest rate of road accident fatality, an inescapable thought as I steered my way along its twisting highways in the direction of East Dereham.

I could tell I was back in rural England because of the low-flying aircraft and because every town seemed to be twinned with somewhere I had never heard of. The many East Anglian air bases could be seen behind mesh fences along the hay-blown roads and in the car stickers that said 'I love F-111s'. Yet as the Dereham GP I had come to visit had discovered through his clinic, some of the bases were a deception. They had been converted into turkey factories whose production lines took thirty minutes to turn a clucking bird into a cutlet. Dr Abell might still be called out to the airforce child whose hand was stuck in a Coke machine but it was the turkey workers and their painful joints who were more often waiting in his surgery.

I hadn't imagined that the turkey trade carried a health hazard but Chris Abell had grown suspicious of the procession of aching wrists and stiff shoulders. Finally he had asked one of his patients what his job entailed.

'He said he was a hanger-on at the bird factory. When the turkeys appear, someone has to hang them on a hook: just that, over and over again, lifting fat birds and hanging them upside down.' Chris believed that men doing this work suffered a kind of repetitive strain injury, a condition so popular it had its own abbreviation, RSI. In the City of London, it was blamed on the over-use of computer keyboards but I would hear about it again the following day from trawlermen, who had known it for years as Jumbo Wrist. In the turkey business, it was said to afflict more than just the hangers-on.

'When the turkeys have been killed and plucked and cut open, someone has to put his hand inside and pull out the intestines so that the vet, who is standing one place along the conveyor belt, can inspect them. And after 22,000 turkeys a day, he gets RSI as well.' Chris was the kind of vegetarian who loved to tell gory tales.

We were strolling through East Dereham and Chris was waving to his patients with the *bonhomie* of someone standing for Parliament. Perhaps it was a habit; he had once been a candidate in a by-election and won 102 votes for the NHS Supporters Party. I had come to his practice to look for clues to East Anglia's good health. Most men and women in Britain will die of heart disease, chest infections or tumours, particularly of the lung and the breast. This is also true in East Anglia, but comparisons with other regions are revealing. Here men have the lowest mortality rate for coronary thrombosis and the second lowest for chronic bronchitis and lung cancer. Women have the lowest rate for all three and the third lowest for breast cancer.

It would be naïve to search for a single key to these happy statistics and even multiple causes were hard to identify and piece together. But the first place to look was the staple diet of epidemiologists: smoking, drinking and the wrong food. No less an observer of Englishmen than J. B. Priestley wrote, 'The East Anglian is a solid man. Lots of beef and beer, tempered with the east wind, have gone into the making of him.' Local surveys bear out the solid image. Forty-eight per cent of East Anglians are judged to be overweight, although this is only a little above the national figure of 44 per cent. But on average, men drink less alcohol here than anywhere else and only 11 per cent of men are counted as heavy drinkers, meaning they consume more than three and a half pints three times a week, compared to 29 per cent in the English North.

And diet? It was hard to believe that the East Anglian was a natural food faddist, pecking at fish oils and bran. But sales of low fat milks were reputedly high and sales of white bread were low, though this might reflect the habits of young people alone. As for tobacco, on which the nation as a whole spends 7 per cent of its income, East Anglians were more self-denying than most, limiting themselves to less than 6 per cent.

What did Chris think of the beef and beer image? He hadn't noticed it – nor the whey and wholemeal alternative. General practice here was like everywhere else – a battle to bring comfort to the homes of the elderly – and the habits of patients seemed not to be unusual. Nor did wealth appear to be the answer. People weren't obviously richer, though as long ago as in the Domesday Book the region's prosperity was being remarked on and though unemployment at the time of my visit was running at half the national rate. In any case, the low mortality was spread across all social classes.

Perhaps good health had been imported. From the late sixteenth century, the Huguenots, fleeing religious persecution, joined other migrants from the lowlands of northern Europe in bringing their weaving skills to Norfolk, a leader in the wool trade. Eventually more than a third of the population of Norwich was foreign. Priestley, visiting in the 1930s, saw the pointed chins on East Anglian faces as a legacy of Flemish immigration. Did the same movement also pass on longevity, which can also be found today in the Low Countries?

It was an appealing story but a thin theory. Just as in the Western Isles there was no one cause of so much heart disease, in East Anglia, where there was relatively little, there was no single explanation that could be pinned down and exported to Britain's high risk cities and islands. Somehow East Anglia's history and habits, its migrants, its land and its genes had been woven together to produce good health in the same way that a winning hand is dealt from a shuffled pack. But you can't say to someone: if you shuffle like this, you'll serve the same hand. And you can't soften the arteries of the Outer Hebrides with a single suggestion, however sweeping. But Chris did have one home-grown explanation, or at least he obligingly invented one.

'Once a year I go to a friend's farm and I work in his beet fields. For a week I plod along rows of beet and think about nothing else . . . just beet. By the time I leave, my mind is completely empty and I feel so relaxed . . .'

'Are you saying it's the pace of life that's healthy?'

When he said yes, he was nearly chuckling; whether at me or himself wasn't clear. It was a favourite urban fantasy, this image of pastoral calm. And this was the medical version: no stress meant less need for alcohol and tobacco, which meant less heart and chest disease. But, as we both knew, as a portrait of modern rural life, with its long-distance commuting, its frustrating traffic and its declining agricultural labour, it belonged with the straw-chewing yokel sitting on the gatepost, predicting the weather. It was an invention. And it ignored the other unexplained superlative to be found in East Anglia's health records, the highest suicide rate in England.

The road on which I headed north to Walsingham was once one of England's busiest highways. So many pilgrims from across Europe took the healing waters that their crowded route was likened to the Milky Way which, under its new name of Walsingham Way, was thought to guide the sick to sanctuary. Then came the Reformation which halted its royal patronage, burned its Virgin and hanged its sub-prior in a field where the railway terminal later stood, until it was converted into the Russian Orthodox Church.

It was in 1061 that a young widowed mother, Richeldis de Favarches, was transported in a vision to Nazareth, where the Mother of God instructed her to build a replica of her Holy House. This she did, near some pagan wells beside the River Stiffkey in Walsingham Parva. Soon the chapel and its waters were renowned for their miraculous powers and frequented by kings and lepers alike.

During the five centuries of Walsingham's glory, leprosy was the most terrifying of curses, regarded like the Eyam plague as a divine punishment for sin just as health was a reward for devotion. Anyone judged by a priest to be infected was given a bell and a begging bowl and forced to live by the roadside, dependent for food on passers-by who had first to be warned to keep their distance. Apart from banishment there was no treatment, although purging and bleeding were sometimes tried, or more commonly a cocktail of boiled adder and leeks; whether as a drink or an ointment, no one now knows.

The last king to visit the shrine was Henry VIII, who came with Catherine of Aragon. But in the ecclesiastical turmoil that followed their divorce, sentiment did not prevent him from tearing down the chapel and martyring its rebellious devotees. A completely unbelievable legend has Henry repenting as he lay dying of neurosyphilis and offering his soul to the Walsingham Virgin.

I parked my car on the site of the old leper hospital and walked to the Anglican shrine, itself a replica of Richeldis's original. On the inside wall, around the main door, there was an uneven tiling of wooden plaques thanking Our Lady of Walsingham for preventing an assortment of calamities, each referring to 'OLW', in the same way that lab workers and junior executives call their boss by his initials.

Some plaques were more calamitous than others. There were those that disguised their despair in hollow optimism, thanking OLW for nothing more miraculous than 'improvement'. Others were more difficult to dismiss as a concoction of faith, like the several that claimed the recovery of sight. One was grateful for help with finance; not, I thought, an area where wonders are often performed. But the date was 1933 and that explained it.

By an unpleasant irony, a shrine attendant I spoke to appeared to be suffering from Alzheimer's dementia, a disease in need of a miracle but which would settle for improvement. Several times he forgot he had already shown me a plaque he thought I'd find interesting; later, while pointing to where the healing was to take place, he couldn't recall the word 'statue'. The plaque was dated 1982 and told of a woman's recovery from brain disease. He said he had seen her recently; she could walk as well as I could. Yes, hers was a miraculous case but no, he didn't know what had been wrong.

The village of Walsingham thrives on an industry of suffering. The Orthodox souvenirs are gaunt icons. In the Catholic shop you can buy St Sebastian pierced by arrows the size of spears. Now I was about to see real suffering as it was sprinkled with Walsingham water. Pilgrims were filing past the Chapel of the Agony in the Garden and, watched by a statue of the Virgin with a massive sword embedded in her heart, heading for the well. Most looked reverent but not ill.

They drank the water, were blessed with it, and took a handful for their own use. A woman in a wheelchair rubbed it into her leg. Someone who was clearly mentally ill wrung his hands with it. In the queue stood a stocky man carrying a child. His T-shirt read ADIS – DON'T DIE OF DYSLEXIA. Here of all places, what would be the reaction to a joke about Aids, a fatal illness as stigmatizing as leprosy itself once was? His turn came and the priest scanned the T-shirt with a solemn lack of understanding. After what I had heard in Edinburgh, I wanted the man to be thrown out. Perhaps the place was making me pious. I left and followed the signs to the Slipper Chapel.

At the peak of the shrine's fame in the Middle Ages the pilgrim road was dotted with chapels, hostelries and some of England's earliest hospitals. After the final stopping point, the journey was completed without shoes. A century ago, the Slipper Chapel was rediscovered by Charlotte Boyd; she had wanted to found an Anglican Order but promptly converted to Catholicism, triggering a small religious feud before the old building could be restored. Now it stands beside the Roman Catholic Church, which was today trumpeting a message of unity and anxiously awaiting the next day's Pentecostal procession, which the previous year had been stormed by Protestant fundamentalists.

On the way there, I came across two modern pilgrims jogging the other way, conspicuous young men with bare feet and a shopping bag, murmuring prayers in unison, boasting of their faith. I didn't stay long. With an open-air mass under way, attendants offered me a place in the line of floral tributes but I declined. I tried to enter the Slipper Chapel but they declined – not while the service was on; but it seemed to be on for ever. Walking back, I met the jogging pilgrims coming the other way, still murmuring.

I had seen faith healing and was prepared to believe it worked. Medicine had hijacked it and built its own replica, calling it the placebo response or the right mental attitude, which research now suggested could prolong life in terminal illness. It was a new idea with a lengthy past.

It also contained an uncomfortable mediaeval echo. Ideas which viewed survival, like good salesmanship, as a product of positive thinking, were not far from seeing people who were too ill to improve as responsible for their condition, like dying pilgrims whose faith must be flawed. In leprosy and Aids certainly, but also in madness, syphilis, addictions, and many others, what was healthy had been too often confused with what was moral.

Yet I was aware that cynicism came on a plate in a place such as Walsingham, with its centuries of *naïveté*, intolerance and honest-to-God malice. That it was awash with icons and graven images was no secret. That most of the health-seeking pilgrims were already healthy should not have been a surprise. What was astonishing was that it was possible to witness such a scene at all.

How had faith healing survived the advent of high-tech medicine? There was a literary answer from Bernard Shaw who, in his introduction to *A Doctor's Dilemma*, put forward his opinion that faith could be produced in any intensity by a simple desire to believe and some sort of pay-off, or words to that effect. There was also an answer from rat psychology where an action that produces occasional, random success will be repeated far more than one which carries a predictable outcome.

And there was an answer in human fear and superstition. Nine hundred years ago, diseases would engulf the body in inexplicable decay, abruptly and without reason. Now, although the causes of illness have names, they are no less puzzling: submicroscopic living particles, molecules that disrupt our genes. And diagnoses are reached through bewildering technology. The incomprehensibility produces fear and fear produces faith.

Even so, it was impossible to leave the shrine without a sense of intrigue that went beyond voyeurism, and a sense of awe that was not just pity. There was something about the crowd at the sprinkling, perhaps the docile way they queued for their miracles, that would leave an observer subdued and tired of feeling sceptical. It was impossible to doubt that, to the pilgrims who were sick or afraid, Walsingham was a vital place. To them it held out a magical straw at which to clutch.

I made one stop on my route to Lowestoft, an attempt to uncover the origins of Britain's most renowned nurse after Florence Nightingale. Edith Cavell had been born in Swardeston, a village a few miles outside Norwich whose cathedral had buried her in its precincts. The roads in that part of Norfolk are double-jointed threads that lead you on an angled, back-tracking path so that you are continually lost. They must be the descendants of much older links between villages, meant to guide local people from one place only as far as the next; perhaps at one time no one was likely to be walking further. Nowadays they never add up to a coherent journey. Lost again, I pulled into a cul-de-sac lined by recent bungalows and tried to trace on my map how I had reached wherever I was. When I looked up, I saw a street sign spelling 'Cavell Road'.

Swardeston turned out to be a rim of not very old houses and a surprisingly large pet shop along a straight half-mile of road. Apart from the church that seemed to be hiding from casual visitors, little of the present village could have existed even fifty years ago, let alone when Edith Cavell was a child here, a decade or so after the Crimean War had given respectability to the profession she would enter. Even the local monument to her was modern.

Where in her early life was the germ of her decision, when almost fifty years old in 1914, to care for the victims of her own war, the mutilated and feverish soldiers of the Belgian trenches? How had her years in this village matured into heroism, leading her to assist the escape of men in her care and then refuse to inform on her accomplices, guaranteeing her execution by German firing-squad? Looking around, I knew the answers were not in present-day Swardeston but the truth was they would not have been in the Swardeston of 1865 either. I had been close to making the biographer's assumption, you could say the psychiatrist's assumption, that there are roots of remarkable acts that can always be found in an unremarkable past. But just as often, and spontaneous courage offered a likely example, there was no logical pattern of predetermination. Outstanding bravery – and for that matter outstanding wickedness – were qualities of ordinary people under extraordinary conditions.

In Lowestoft there was a harbour to see but only remnants of its mighty fishing fleets, tucked behind warehouses at the end of an industrial road, as if the town itself had turned its back on its trawling past. It must have been near here that Daniel Defoe dipped his toe in the water, just as he did at each coastal extremity.

Across the deck of the *Clarinda H* was a tangle of wet rope which called for wary walking. The crew, or two of them, had just finished ripping out the net that had seized their rudder at sea the previous day; it had forced them to return home before the end of the usual twelve-day stretch, trawling for 'anything', as they put it, mainly plaice. A smell of used oil had settled in the galley, a narrow room lined by a bench on one side and a sink and a cooker on the other, connected to the outside air by an opaque porthole. On the small table a shallow Fray Bentos tin had seen long service as an ash-tray. From the wall a calendar model pouted at us like a fish. It was here that Hutch, the captain of the *Clarinda H*, told me what I wanted to know about Dogger Bank itch.

A few months earlier I had come across the itch in a monstrous textbook of medicine. It was a tome of several million words but only a few lines were given over to this curious dermatitis which, it seemed, was an occupational disease of North Sea fishermen. No further reference was provided and I could find no mention of it anywhere else, not even in a huge gruesome atlas of skin disease. I became suspicious while arranging my trip to Lowestoft when the name of the ailment was treated with incredulity by people who ought to have known about it. Perhaps I was the latest victim of a fisherman's yarn which generations of gullible medics had swallowed.

But the reverse was true. Dogger Bank itch was a contact eczema notorious among trawlermen. Many had seen their skin grow cracked and painful enough to drive them from their jobs, often with puny compensation, though the luckier ones were able to transfer to deep sea fishing, which was less abrasive. The men who worked the North Sea knew all about Dogger Bank itch and it was doctors who thought it was rare.

Its cause was curly weed, a pale brown, waterlogged seaweed common in shallow seas and so in abundance around the Dogger Bank, where it multiplied in the warmer water of spring and summer. In the indiscriminate mechanics of trawling it was dragged up in the nets and from there it smeared any skin that came near the catch. After one outbreak the skin was sensitized and needed only minimal contact with the weed, even the touch of an empty net, to flare up again. One man Hutch could remember was left besieged by his ultrasensitivity. 'His house faced out to sea. If he opened his front door and there was an easterly wind, his rash would come back.'

Hutch wore a stout boiler-suit from which emerged meaty hands and a convivial neck. He spoke in short, deliberate sentences and during his frequent pauses the other crew member nodded and winked at me. He had a favourite story about the amusing ignorance of doctors. It concerned someone who was tortured by Dogger Bank itch every year from March to October. Within minutes his rash might erupt until a prickly inflammation covered his whole body except for his back. But, said Hutch, he was a man with connections. 'His friends were educated people. They told him to see a private doctor.'

So he did, and brought with him a piece of curly weed which was soon taped to his back along with several other potential irritants. By the next appointment, the place where the weed had been attached was an excoriated mess. The specialist was triumphant. 'I know what's wrong. It's Dogger Bank itch,' he announced. But Hutch's friend knew that already. He also knew his back would no longer be spared. And that there was no treatment.

While we were talking, two men from another boat entered, carrying a broad bucket overflowing with live lobsters, and placed it, slightly incongruously, beside the microwave. Hutch asked if they had ever suffered any fishermen's illnesses. One said, 'Fish fever,' and everyone laughed, including me. Then Hutch thought of jumbo wrist, a tendon injury from repeated gutting, a jumbo being a 3 pound haddock. Today it is caused by eviscerating plaice; the crew of some of the larger vessels may have to slit over 100,000 on return to port. There were other hazards, with names like haddock rash, fish erysipeloid, and tit-juice conjunctivitis. What was fish fever, I wanted to know. More laughter, but not as loud.

Fish fever is an ecstasy of fishermen whose nets are brimming. Only once, while trawling the freezing water off Norway, had Hutch felt its intoxicating presence. The *Clarinda H* had spent a miserable ten days at sea. Although she was due back in Lowestoft within 48 hours, her hold was empty and her crew fatigued. Suddenly, dramatically, the nets filled and filled again. No sooner were they dropped than they were hauled up, alive and spilling over. All day long the decks were frantic with success. The time came and went when the boat should have pointed homewards but a euphoric Hutch would not leave. 'Deadlines are important. You have to be back on time. But it was a real big catch. I couldn't stop.' Eventually his men confronted him and persuaded him to call his feast enough.

If there was a biblical sound to fish fever, it was in keeping with how the sea itself was spoken of, like a punishing deity, a provider of miracles but irascible, demanding sacrifice. And it was no wonder that it was viewed this way because the greatest threat to the health of fishermen was the sea itself.

Fishing boats were among the most dangerous of workplaces, injuring and drowning their crew through the combined force of heaving seas and heavy equipment. As a vessel rolled in the swell, an unlucky man could be struck by an unstable load or a swinging hook. Simmering pots could be tossed across anyone standing near the stove. I heard the story of someone who fell from the mast while, of all things, trying to change a light bulb.

The worst fear was the fear of capsizing. There are places around Iceland where the rigging becomes glazed with ice that forms too quickly and too thickly to remove, until the top-heavy boat has a menacing sway. Still more dreadful is the instability induced by the method of fishing itself. Many trawlers have huge metal rods on each side and from these are hung the nets which scrape along the sea bed collecting mud, rocks and weed as well as fish. This can add up to such a weight that the solid rods are bent 'like bananas', as the favoured simile goes. That, though, is not the problem. The problem occurs when only one of the nets is clogged with mud because, as the craft tries to move forward or, worse, pull up its catch, the imbalance can tip it over.

Some years ago, Hutch trailed one net through a bank of silt and he still tells what happened next in the careless tone that some people use to describe misery or terror. First the *Clarinda H* listed and veered to one side, then it began a slow spin. Out of control and partly up-ended, it could have rolled over at any second. The order to abandon ship was immediate.

The North Sea is no one's idea of a hostess. Once the lifeboats were lowered, they lurched and swung on its surface. For their occupants these were perilous minutes but, despite their own insecurity, all eyes were on the danger they had just left. On the bridge they could see the captain struggling with his ship which was now turning foolish circles.

If you ask someone what happened when he was at the point of death or during an act of startling self-sacrifice, what did he think about or discover, what personal limits did he cross, the answer is always mundane and can amount to literally nothing. The moment arises, action is taken or perhaps not, then it passes. There is no clairvoyance, no calculation of risk, odds or the meaning of survival, and no nod in the direction of mortality. It can seem an amazing contradiction, a disappointment even, a missed opportunity at a peak of endurance. But it could be what makes such a peak possible. Hutch stayed on board. The spinning stopped and the list diminished. The crew climbed back and the nets were gently raised.

With stresses like this, no further excuse is needed for the prodigious drinking of men whose job is the sea. The drunken sailor, the spliced mainbrace and the rum-sodden sea-dog are part of a seafaring culture in which alcoholism is routine. Deaths from liver cirrhosis follow an occupational pattern with high rates in three crude groups. There are those who work with drink: barmen, publicans, chefs and hoteliers. There are those whose trade is oiled by drink, such as company directors and journalists. And there are the others, the fishermen, sailors, doctors and financiers, not obviously related unless by the alleged stress of how they earn their bread and their brandy.

Fishermen are reputedly binge-drinkers, a result of having brass in pocket and not very long to blow it. They may have only two or three days on shore but the wages and the thirst of two weeks' hard labour. Losing both used to be as easy as falling off a bar-stool, as trawling towns were lined by countless drinking dens.

Once back at sea, the shakes of alcohol withdrawal were, still are, a well-known nuisance but serious only if an omen of delirium tremens, the DTs, a terrifying state of confusion, hallucinations and paranoia. Difficult enough to control in a hospital ward, it is hard to imagine how it could have been coped with on a fishing-boat, except by administering more rum.

Hutch thought it was rarely seen now and that even rarer was continued drinking once the anchor had been weighed. It simply was not allowed and everyone complied because everyone knew the sense of it. While he told me this, his partner went on winking but I knew the skipper was correct. In fact, just once did Hutch tell me something that left me doubtful. As I was leaving I asked how long he had been a fisherman. All his working life, he replied, a total of more than thirty years, although for two years he gave it up.

'Why was that?' I wanted to know. I wondered what secret he would tell me, what piece of his life was hidden in the two-year gap. But Hutch simply looked straight at me and said with finality: 'I didn't like it.'

Suffolk began to look like Essex as I headed south. Beet fields gave way to sugar refineries, two-car driveways to second-hand showrooms. East Anglia's population was known to be multiplying, partly with a Hampstead overspill (you could see signs outside cottages: 'Fresh eggs – raspberries – picture framing') and partly with Londoners looking for work. Driving in this direction was like watching the growth on fast forward.

The village of Bures straddles the River Stour, with the Suffolk parish of Bures St Mary linked by a narrow bridge to its Essex twin, Bures Hamlet. In this corner of England, John Constable haunts every tea-room and boarding-house. But the landscape around Bures is less likely to own up to its medical connection as the exporter of a notorious disease and, in the same breath, a persecutor of witches.

Centre stage at the story's denouement stands George Huntington, an American physician, who at the end of his career in 1910 told the New York Neurological Society of a portentous incident from his boyhood on Long Island more than fifty years earlier:

> Driving with my father through a wooded road leading from East Hampton to Amagansetl, we suddenly came upon two women, mother and daughter, both tall, thin, almost cadaverous, both bowing, twisting, grimacing. I stared in wonderment, almost in fear. What could it mean? My father paused to speak with them and we passed on.

It was his first encounter with the condition which is still known as Huntington's chorea. In 1872 he described its classic features: its appearance for the first time in adult life, its slow, unremitting course, direct transmission from parent to offspring, and failure to recur once the line of transmission has been broken. Since then it has been found to be a disorder of the brain's basal ganglia, marked by chorea (the writhing and twitching Huntington witnessed as a boy) and mental signs from behavioural disturbance to psychosis to dementia.

It is unusual in that, although directly inherited, it often does not become manifest until around the age of forty and here lies the secret of its persistence because, by the time a carrier is known to have the illness, it has already been passed on to half his or her children. This powerful pattern of heredity has also placed Huntington's chorea at the centre of current research into the molecular genetics of inherited disorders. It is now known to be transmitted as an abnormality of chromosome 4 and a biochemical test can identify those who carry the defective chromosome before the clinical illness becomes apparent. This has the important advantage of allowing someone to know he or she has nothing to fear or, if the result is bad, at least to make an informed decision whether or not to have children who will each carry a 50 per cent risk. In fact, many prefer uncertainty to taking the test, having seen a parent deteriorate and die.

To George Huntington, studying chorea was a family business. His father and grandfather were both doctors and they had observed the strange hereditary disease of movements and madness which drove some victims to suicide. They knew that it was common in the vicinity of East Hampton, although reports of geographical clusters had also come from other parts of the United States.

George's grandfather, Abel Huntington, had moved to East Hampton in 1797 and his father, George Lee, lived there all his life. It was a town which English immigrants had built, initially naming it Maidstone when settling there in 1649. Many of those who reached New England, including large numbers who were seeking to take their Puritanism to the New World, had come from East Anglia. One such person was Simon Huntington, forebear of the Long Island medical men, who with his family left Norwich in 1633 and sailed from Great Yarmouth aboard the *Elizabeth Bonaventure*. A fellow passenger was Thomas Lincoln, a weaver from Hingham, believed to have been an ancestor of the sixteenth US president.

Three years before that, two brothers, William and Nicholas Knapp, of the parish of Bures St Mary, travelled to Southampton, boarded one of a group of ships known as the Winthrop fleet and journeyed to Boston Bay; John Winthrop, a lawyer from Groton near Bures, became Governor there. Scholars still argue passionately over the minutiae of the Knapp genealogy, which is shrouded by a haze of pseudonyms, misleading references and antiquity. Yet it remains likely that the Knapps took with them the gene for Huntington's chorea, which then spread throughout North America.

Not that the choreic movements were then recognized as such. This was a time of great excitement over witchcraft both in puritanical East Anglia and in the New World colonies, a time of accusations, of trial by ordeal. Nor was a belief in witches simply a product of ignorance or religious frenzy. Sir Thomas Browne, the seventeenth-century author who also practised as a doctor in Norwich, referred to it in his writing.

The body of knowledge surrounding witchcraft included details that meant trouble for people with certain illnesses, chorea among them. To the skin and nipples of witches it was thought that imps attached themselves, causing fits and weird motions of the body, and possession by animals was betrayed in the same way. It was said that twitching and writhing were a satanic mockery of Christ's agony on the cross. Disturbed behaviour which was really the product of a malfunctioning brain could be construed as wilful immorality. Some sufferers would have developed religious delusions and it is not hard to see how unfortunate choreics might run into a charge of witchcraft which they might even believe themselves.

Whatever else was rife in the Knapp family, they shared a knack of falling foul of authority. As soon as they landed in New England, Nicholas – said to be a vendor of medicines – was fined five shillings for selling expensive, useless water to fellow travellers who had been sick with scurvy. William, meanwhile, seems to have spent a good deal of his first few years in America under arrest for an assortment of petty crimes, such as public profanity, selling beer without a licence and making an offensive speech against Governor Winthrop.

How much of this was attributable to chromosome 4 can only be guessed. Probably none of it. But what happened from then on is another matter. One of William's sons was charged with 'distemper' and another died prematurely in squalor. A third likewise died young in 1658, but not before marrying Elizabeth Warne and producing a daughter, also called Elizabeth. His widow returned, with her new husband John Buttery, to Bures where their family grew but fears of evil spirits pursued them. Once, during a quarrel, one of their children suffered a convulsion which Buttery accused his wife of bringing on through sorcery. By the law of the time, he was entitled to lock her in gaol until she confessed and this she did after three days and nights.

What then happened to her is uncertain, but not so what befell her daughter Elizabeth, the grandchild of William Knapp. She found fame as the 'Groton witch', known for the violent contortions of her body. But it was a daughter of William who most infuenced the chorea story when she moved to East Hampton, Long Island. There she became the source of the many cases who in the nineteenth century would inspire three generations of doctors called Huntington.

The Knapp lineage is complicated by the fate of Nicholas's wife Ellin who, although not a blood relative, was charged with witchcraft and hanged in 1653. It was a reminder that, as with Elizabeth Warne, it was not only by harbouring the wrong genes that you could find fingers pointing your way.

Her execution exposed how dangerous it was to oppose religious or political authority. As Ellin stepped towards the gallows, she appeared to whisper to Roger Ludlow, the Deputy Governor of Massachussetts and Connecticut, who was there to see his version of justice performed. Then, facing the noose, she allowed the public ceremony to proceed. Within a few minutes, her lifeless body had been cut down so that spectators could examine it for the tell-tale sucking marks. Heads were already nodding when a young woman called Mary Staplies declared, in a voice that hurled blame at Ludlow, that there were none. 'If Ellin was a witch,' cried Mary, 'then I too am a witch.'

This brave outburst permitted Ludlow to reply that she was indeed possessed and that Ellin had told him so moments before her death. Mary was lucky. Her husband promised to sue the Deputy Governor if he ever repeated the slander and for a time nothing more came of their animosity. Years later, however, in 1692 – the year of the celebrated witch trials in Old Salem – the accusation finally caught up with Mary, when she was tried along with her daughter and granddaughter. Once again her luck held and all three were set free. Also that year, the granddaughter of Ellin and Nicholas Knapp, a renowned eccentric named Mercy Didsborough, was twice pronounced innocent of the same crime.

One of Nicholas's daughters married the son of someone whose name has been quoted as Jeffers but who may have been Jeffrey Knapp, a half-brother to William and Nicholas. Both partners being possible carriers, they had no difficulty in passing on the disorder to their descendants. Meanwhile, Jeffrey's remaining sons met with mixed fortunes. Ironically, one sat on the jury at one of Mercy Didsborough's trials. Two more were choreic and one of these was found guilty of 'bestiality' as a young man. His punishment was to be fined, flogged, flogged again and made to wear a halter for two years. When it was removed he not surprisingly left New England and is believed to have scattered his genes throughout the country. Many of the pockets of chorea across the map of America were probably the result of his adventures.

Wandering around the churchyard of Bures St Mary, I turned over the unanswered question in the saga. If a family from this village took Huntington's chorea over the Atlantic, how before that did it reach here? Chroniclers tracing back the Knapp ancestry find the trail dries up in Bures though no one believes the disease had just arisen from a new genetic mutation. It was the ideal vacuum for speculation and what had stirred my imagination was another account of chorea spreading to the New World, this time to Newfoundland.

It concerns a brother and sister, Georges and Marie, whose surname has been lost. They were Huguenots who lived near the French-Swiss border until the revocation of the Edict of Nantes forced them to seek a fresh home. Their flight led them to Nova Scotia and their families later settled in Colchester County on its northern coast. Mary had six children, four of whom became choreic, as did twelve of her twenty-one grandchildren and fifteen of her twenty-nine great-grandchildren. For many years the disease in that part of Canada was confined to Colchester County.

Could it be that, in the sixteenth century, during a previous phase of Huguenot migration, the Huntington gene travelled to East Anglia at the same time that Flemish weavers and other traders thronged the region? If so, it would bring a final pathos to the tale of witches and twitches. Because, in escaping one form of religious persecution, the Huguenots may have spread the seed of another.

TWELVE

Central London

AT THE north end of Harley Street you can turn your back on the bustle of Marylebone Road and gaze along a line of arched doorways and brass plates, the outer crust of medicine's private world. It is a street that has grown rich on snobbery and second opinions, a glossy spot that some doctors still aspire to, waiting for the day when their chance might come to occupy *rooms*.

Harley Street seemed a good place to begin exploring central London but it was not somewhere to linger. London was where I had come to pick up the threads of the stories I had encountered throughout the country, to rediscover the characters who had peopled my medical journey, to follow the plots of their lives and find out what happened next. All roads had led me eventually to the capital and it was here that I anticipated tying up at least a few of the many loose ends. And Harley Street I wanted to see not only because it represents the monied end of medicine but because of Florence Nightingale.

A year before Britain entered the Crimean War Florence too passed through Harley Street. She had been appointed in 1853 as Superintendant of the Institution for the Care of Sick Gentlewomen in Distressed Circumstances, having impressed Lady Canning at interview with her 'quiet sensible manner'. Although such a view of her character was in a minority, as most people saw her as a harridan, Elizabeth Gaskell also gave a favourable account of her disposition, describing her as fun and a skilled mimic. Florence, however, mocked the institution as a 'Sanitarium for Sick Governesses run by a Committee of Fine Ladies' and accepted the job only on the condition that she would be given absolute authority.

The institution was sited at 90 Harley Street and one of Florence's first achievements was to harangue the committee of fine ladies until they provided her with *rooms* nearby, at number 1. Next she sacked the entire staff, including a doctor – a daring move in those hierarchical days – and replaced them with people she preferred. She also imposed a two-month limit on the time patients could stay there, arguing that otherwise they had 'no incentive to get well', although she made an exception of those who were dying. She was, after all, the future Lady with the Lamp.

By January 1854, less than a year after taking up her post, she was bored and looking for excitement elsewhere. She assisted in a surgical operation using Simpson's new anaesthetic gas, chloroform. She volunteered to help out at the Middlesex Hospital, whose wards were being overwhelmed by the latest epidemic of cholera. The institution she had transformed she now referred to as a 'little mole-hill'; the Crimean War was the stage she needed.

Number 90 Harley Street sports one of London's ubiquitous blue plaques, celebrating the history of the city. It records only that Florence Nightingale left for Crimea from that address. Number 1 is now a solicitor's office. It was not a doctor but a nurse who was the most famous practitioner from Harley Street but there was little in this line of private clinics to comemmorate her. I turned into Cavendish Square, rejoined the crowds and the traffic and headed for Soho.

Crossing Oxford Circus and walking down Carnaby Street I reached Broadwick Street. Running across the centre of Soho, it connects the souvenir shops and leather stores in the west of the district to the recording studios, film company headquarters and eating joints in the east. In 1854, under its previous name of Broad Street, it was dirty, cramped and ridden with disease. Like Bolton during the same period, it crammed its too many residents into too little space. Whole families lived in one room, the average number to a house was eighteen and there was even a house that could boast fifty-four occupants. The conditions were ideal for the spread of diseases, including cholera.

As the plague had done in Dorset, cholera had arrived in Britain by boat, only this time it had been a northern port, Sunderland, that had first experienced it, during 1831. By the next year it had reached

Edinburgh and then other large towns and the first epidemic of the disease had been witnessed. Over the subsequent twenty years outbreaks in cities such as London were regular events and public health measures such as improvement in sanitation were being advocated by Edwin Chadwick, Lord Shaftesbury and the latter's colleague in assessing the health of children in the coal-mines, Dr Southwood Smith. But the cause of cholera remained unknown, although contemporary theories had linked it to malodorous air and river water.

Enter John Snow, the doctor who legitimized chloroform by administering it to Queen Victoria during the birth of Prince Leopold. Unlike most of the medical profession at the time Snow was drawn to the river water theory and aware too of the easy spread of the disease in overcrowded conditions. He pondered over the part played by poor toilet facilities and he hypothesized that a person might become infected by swallowing something – 'a peculiar poison or morbid matter' – from a cholera victim. These ideas he was able to combine in a novel notion of water-borne and (as it is now called) faecal–oral spread. If someone with cholera contaminated his bed sheets with diarrhoea, whoever was nursing him could not avoid touching the infective material. If that individual was then in contact with food eaten by the rest of the household – and in the crowded rooms of Soho this seemed inevitable – the disease would quickly spread. Cholera-infested faeces could also seep into the wells from which drinking water was drawn or into the rivers that fed the wells and street pumps.

Snow's opportunity to confirm his ideas came during the 1854 epidemic in the affair of the Broad Street pump. Having arrived in the capital in 1853 as part of a national outbreak, cholera killed thousands of inhabitants of central London within a year. From 31 August 1854 there was a sudden acceleration in the rate of deaths in Soho, particularly in and around Broad Street. In the street itself there was a victim in thirty-seven of forty-nine houses and in the immediate surroundings no fewer than 344 people died in the first four days of September.

Water from the pump in Broad Street was widely held to be tastier than what could be obtained elsewhere in the district and some residents of distant burghs even sent to Soho for a supply. A local sherbert shop and several coffee houses used it in their recipes. It was the owner of one such coffee shop who alerted Snow to what was happening in the area when she wrote to him on 6 September with the information that nine of her customers had died in the previous few days.

Snow's suspicions immediately fell on the pump, although those who believed in bad air as the means of spread blamed the foul drains for the outbreak. Others blamed emanations from the old Plague Pit in Little Marlborough Street at a site where one of London's more glamorous stores now stands. But the water emitted from the pump must have told Snow he was right. Far from being the stuff people would send servants across the city to collect, it was now stinking. Snow examined eighty-three of the Soho deaths from the first few days of September and found seventy-three to live in the immediate vicinity of the pump, sixty-one of whom were known to draw their water from it. Of the other ten, five more victims lived in adjacent streets and, although it was not their closest source, preferred to walk to Broad Street because of the superior quality of its water. Three were children attending a school nearby and would have used the pump regularly. The remaining two were people who lived further away, one in Hampstead where there was otherwise no cholera, and who had the Broad Street effluent specially delivered.

Convinced now that water carried the morbid matter responsible for the disease, Snow went on to carry out research that is still talked of with misty-eyed awe by epidemiologists. He compared the incidence of cholera in different districts, streets and even rows of houses and found the rates to vary according to the water company providing the supply.

Two of the largest providers of water to central London, the Southwark and Vauxhall Water Company and the Lambeth Water Company, supplied roughly the same areas through pipes that ran together. Both used the Thames as their source. But a few years earlier the Lambeth Water Company had positioned its inlet pipes further upstream than its Southwark and Vauxhall rival, at a greater distance from the outpourings of over three hundred city sewers. Having found out how many houses in total were supplied by each company and whose water was being used in each house where there was a death, Snow calculated the mortality rate from cholera for each water company. The Southwark and Vauxhall Company came out badly, the death rate from its downstream supply being several times higher. Snow not only concluded that water carried cholera, he also speculated that his hypothesized morbid matter was alive and able to multiply in its chosen milieu.

Snow's findings backed up the view of Chadwick and Shaftesbury that the health of the public depended on clean water and efficient waste disposal. And it was Shaftesbury's name that was attached to the airy highway constructed when some of the more insanitary parts of Soho were finally demolished in the late nineteenth century. Recognition of Chadwick was more grudging, being confined in this area to a short street near the Thames. Perhaps this was because Chadwick was by all accounts a cantankerous autocrat, while Shaftesbury managed to be more diplomatic when criticizing governments. Lord John Russell said of him that if he ever took orders he would make him a bishop.

Between Broadwick Street and Shaftesbury Avenue I made my way down Great Windmill Street where, among the hair salons and the Asian restaurants, one of Soho's better known industries still thrives, or at least exists. This is the land of peep shows, etched permanently on the itinerary of out-of-town youths who arrive in groups to nudge and yell at each other. But to the majority of people who walk down them, streets like this are simply short cuts from theatre to dining table or pub to pub; they are too busy going somewhere else to notice the slice of Old England that they are passing through. 'Explicit,' said the fluorescent signs: 'Peep Show £1', a price that seemed not to have changed in years. Voyeuristic sex had proved more resistant to inflation than any commodity I could think of. Linger near a Soho doorway for only a second and someone on a cash-till will invite you in. It seemed so old-fashioned I felt almost nostalgic for adolescence.

Beyond the clubs on Great Windmill Street is the back end of the Lyric Theatre, where the medical teaching of William Hunter is celebrated with another blue plaque. In the eighteenth century Hunter dissected, researched and taught where the theatre stands, his lessons attended not only by a generation of budding doctors but by society figures such as Edward Gibbon and Adam Smith. Laymen like these frequented his anatomy classes with the same spirit that some spectators now take to a West End play.

Having initially decided on a career in the Church Hunter took up medicine under the tutelage of Alexander Monro, the founder of a dynasty of Edinburgh anatomists of the same name. From 1720 until 1846 three generations of Alexander Monros were Professors of Anatomy, the grandson being the man who dissected William Burke. Hunter left for London in 1740 and studied for two years in the anatomy school of James Douglas, remembered in medical circles for the pouch of Douglas, a recess behind the uterus. When Douglas died Hunter took over his teaching and from 1746 gave private lectures from premises in Covent Garden.

Anatomy teaching in the early part of the century had been restricted by a combination of the law and rivalry within the medical profession. Dissection had been limited by Parliament to four executed criminals a year, cut up publicly in the hall of the Barber-Surgeons Company. Members of the Company were anxious to preserve their monopoly and prevent the opening of private anatomy schools and for a time they were successful. But in 1745 they came up against an interest more powerful than their own. The government, with future wars in mind, wanted more and better surgeons for the army and so removed the privilege of the barber-surgeons and abolished the quota on suitable corpses.

Private schools sprang up throughout London and in some other cities, especially Edinburgh, and surgeons advertised their tuition in popular newspapers. But the supply of bodies remained a problem. Unseemly scenes could be witnessed after an execution as doctors running their own courses jostled with officials from the Barber-Surgeons Company, each claiming the criminal's remains as theirs. As the number of students and schools went on increasing, resurrection provided the solution.

William Hunter's school in Covent Garden became the most famous in England and every decent student, as well as many members of London society, thronged to its classes. In 1766 new premises were sought, and built at 16 Windmill Street, complete with lecture theatre, dissecting room and stables. Hunter was one of the leading doctors of his day, a friend to artists and aristocrats and the man who delivered the future King George IV, an experience that must have helped him write his chief scientific paper on the structure of the pregnant uterus. He also collaborated with his brother John in publishing on the absorption of lymph and the anatomy of the testis and the tear duct. There were, however, those who doubted the originality of much of his work, including his old mentor Alexander Monro, Monro *fils* and Percival Pott, the doctor who described cancer of the scrotum in chimney sweeps before it also appeared in mulespinners.

Although not the teacher of anatomy his brother was, John Hunter was probably the greater doctor if the breadth of subjects he wrote about is a guide. Ulcers, inflammation, wounds caused by explosions, the structure of the placenta, the muscles in the walls of blood vessels – John Hunter described them all. And then there was 'The Case of Mr Appleby, who had an abscess formed in the gall bladder which opened into the gut, and also externally', the earliest example of a cholecystocolic fistula, a hole into the intestine made by an inflamed gall bladder. In Mr Appleby's case, erosion also occurred through the wall of the abdomen and Hunter was able to observe the abscess discharging on to the surface of the skin and even gallstones emerging into the outside world. His vigour in carrying out experiments was renowned enough for the story to circulate that his angina was caused by syphilitic inflammation of his coronary arteries, the result of inoculating his own penis with infected material for some scientific purpose. There is no doubt that this was untrue, although he did suffer from angina according to Edward Jenner who diagnosed it, and he often took the waters at Bath as treatment. Perhaps someone had confused Jenner the inoculator of cowpox with Hunter the expert on inflammation.

Great men populated his list of patients. David Hume attended him in 1775 because of the swollen liver that killed him the following year. He applied a salt water poultice to the infected neck of Thomas

Gainsborough, though he too subsequently died. Haydn's nose and Byron's club foot were both examined by him – he also vaccinated Byron – and he treated and wrote about his brother William's kidney stones. That he cut a distinguished figure in Georgian society was confirmed when Sir Joshua Reynolds painted his portrait, a professional act he was able to repay in 1792 when he performed the artist's post-mortem. Reynolds, he wrote, had a liver weighing 11 pounds, a tripling in size brought about by cirrhosis.

The anatomy school in Windmill Street continued to prosper after William Hunter's death, having passed into the hands of his nephew Matthew Baillie, another outstanding teacher and a physician to George III. This was the period of resurrectionism, as rampant in London as it was in Edinburgh, and here too there were few questions asked about the source of the cadavers. From 1809 to 1815 one of the lecturers was Peter Mark Roget, whose thesaurus must surely have begun with acceptable synonyms for 'body-snatcher'.

Roget's medical connections were unorthodox. He had been born in Broad Street in Soho; his cousin Sophie had been one of the first people to be vaccinated by Edward Jenner; and he had himself caught typhus from a patient while studying at Edinburgh's Royal Infirmary. His observation that butchers and fishermen did not suffer their share of consumption was the subject of his first scientific paper, published by Thomas Beddoes, Bristol's expert on the illness whose own experiments with gases had been carried out on other men of letters. He was seventy before he started working on his thesaurus but it was not his only non-medical project. He wrote about optics and electricity. He constructed a kind of slide rule and developed logarithmic scales for it. He contributed a chess column to the *Illustrated London News* and designed a miniature chess set. At one point in his career he prepared a report for the government on London's water supply. He could not have predicted that the public pump in the street where he was born would have more impact than anything he could say.

It was not so much the Burke and Hare scandal and a similar case in London that led to the rapid decline of Hunter's school and its closure in 1833. It was the opening of anatomy schools linked closely to teaching hospitals that condemned private tuition in dissection. The subject was taken over once again by the medical establishment and private lectures disappeared quickly from the social scene. The building in Great Windmill Street became a printing works, later a billiard hall, a restaurant and finally a theatre. Now the place where it stood is merely a street to glance at and leave behind. As I left, a few youthful tourists were still hovering near the sex shows, hoping for another sort of anatomy lesson, and I plunged back into the West End crowds and traffic jams.

London is chaos. Its traffic is insane, immobile and angry, its crowds a fast and tireless swell. Side-streets are snarled up from early morning; the city centre is packed and noisy well after midnight. I like the way you can buy Sunday newspapers on Saturday night, as if London is moving by its own high-energy clock. The people, the old streets, the cars and the lights draw you in and wrap you in their inescapable, entangled mayhem. I ignored the traffic signals, dashed across Coventry Street and jumped aside as a van missed me by an inch.

In London my stories from around the country were becoming jumbled; characters were criss-crossing and reappearing in each other's biographies. Snow, Beddoes, Jenner, Shaftesbury had come together like players in the final act of a West End production. Chloroform, body-snatching and cesspits had started as incidents and continued as themes; and there were more connections to come as I headed towards Pall Mall. It was near here that Aneurin Bevan, whose origins I had found to be knocked down, bribed the top brass among hospital doctors into accepting his National Health Service. 'I stuffed their mouths with gold,' he boasted. It was near here also that Henry VIII, who had torn down the Walsingham shrine that marked the end of the lepers' pilgrimage, built St James's Palace using the stone from a local home for 'leprous virgins'. It was here too that Thomas Sydenham, of the battling, puritanical Sydenham family of Dorset, lived and practised medicine.

Sydenham moved to London in 1655, during Oliver Cromwell's period in office, taking a house off King Street, adjacent to Pall Mall. His patients were resident in the area round St James's Park which was then a swamp, not the duck pond it is now. The putrid air above its water was thought to be responsible for fevers, hence the word 'malaria', and it was this that provided Sydenham with most of his business as well as his pioneering ideas.

Meanwhile events were hotting up for his brother William, the Roundhead colonel who by this time had a new job demanding diplomacy rather than the ferocity that had made his name. Cromwell had decided to set up a second parliamentary chamber after the cruel treatment of a Quaker, James Naylor, by a special committee of the Commons, and he had appointed William Sydenham to lead it. Naylor had faced up to the committee with such obscene contempt – John Locke, watching, thought he was mad – that he had been flogged, branded, and 'bored through the tongue'. The Lord Protector thought the Commons needed to be curbed in case it again overstepped the mark, particularly in disputes with him, and a second chamber seemed the answer. But after Cromwell's death, such was the extent of the plotting and intrigue in which Colonel Sydenham immersed himself that eventually he was not only dismissed but barred from holding public office at all. In 1661, after the Restoration of Charles II, William returned to Dorset and, despite being looked after by Thomas, soon died there.

Sydenham was no longer a name to boost a man's political career and anti-Royalist sentiments were not now in fashion. Thomas dropped his remaining political activities and settled instead for being a doctor. He moved his premises round the corner to Pall Mall and opened his doors to the nobility who flocked to the area once the monarchy was back. Only during 1665, the year of the Great Plague that spread to and slaughtered most of Eyam, did he desert London, as did most of his paying customers. Otherwise the rest of his life was spent studying disease in general and central London's fevers in particular. He wrote the works that transformed medicine in Britain, turning it from a mass of superstition into a science based on observation, and classifying its disorders into distinct types. The next generation of doctors, including John Radcliffe, the luminary who in an ungentlemanly moment put a toad in the spa at Bath, were strongly influenced by his methods. The masterly accounts of clinical signs used in medical teaching during the next two hundred and fifty years began with his emphasis on observation as the root of everything. Sherlock Holmes would never have existed without him.

Like Hippocrates, but unlike anyone since, Sydenham studied the natural history of illnesses, not just their symptoms but their progression, and used what he found as the basis of his classification. Fevers, he wrote after fifteen years of watching and treating them in 1676, could be either continued or intermittent; or they could be smallpox. Continued fevers in seventeenth-century London would have included typhus and typhoid but not cholera, which would not appear for over one hundred and fifty years, while the classic intermittent fever was malaria. Smallpox he fittingly placed in a class of its own. It was so common that Sydenham believed it could be a phase in the changing properties of ageing blood.

By convention the treatment of smallpox was to heat the already feverish patients, feeding them hot liquids and wrapping them in steaming cloths. It was Sydenham's opinion that these methods, far from curing anybody, made death even more likely and that it was cooling treatment that patients needed. The old theories of medicine, he wrote, 'have as much to do with treating sick men as the painting of pictures had to do with the sailing of ships'; he dismissed the ministrations of his contemporaries as meddling. Leading doctors of the day retaliated, attacking his methods and calling him a 'western bumpkin' but patients knew whom to trust and consultations with him were highly prized. John Locke wrote a poem praising him. The first Earl of Shaftesbury, his former colleague in the Dorset militia and the ancestor of the nineteenth-century protector of public health, asked many doctors whether he should remove a silver tube that he had had inserted surgically to drain a liver abscess. Views varied but when Sydenham told him to keep it in, he did, wearing it for the rest of his life. As a result a turncock on a large wine jar became known as a Shaftesbury while his political opponents also remarked on it, saying that the drain was too narrow to let out all his corruption.

The list of subjects covered by Sydenham multiplied. Gout, rheumatic fever, pneumonia, pleurisy, quinsy (abscesses around the tonsils) and erysipelas (an infection of the skin) were all depicted in what he wrote, as were a variety of novel therapies. Having cooled smallpox victims, he gave quinine to patients with the ague, the old name for malaria, which is still treated with quinine derivatives; and he gave liquid laudanum, an opiate, for severe pain. But when he thought his patients did not need drugs, he broke with the practice of apothecaries and said so, recommending exercise, fresh air and mineral waters. To feverish patients, many of whom would be dehydrated, he gave fluids including beer, and by this simple measure must have saved many lives.

In suggesting some of these cures, he knew what he was talking about from personal experience. He was over fifty when he published his most important work. Since his twenties he had suffered from gout and kidney stones and had spent weeks at a time on his back in the Earl of Shaftesbury's house. To ease the pain of bumpy coach rides he would consume a quantity of beer before setting out and to help him sleep despite his gouty feet and renal colic he regularly took eighteen drops of laudanum on going to bed.

In his last treatise, produced in 1686, he went on borrowing from personal knowledge of illness by writing about kidney stones and he also identified a distinct form of fever in what may have been the first specific account of typhoid. In the same publication he discussed chorea, the involuntary writhing movements that as a hereditary disease was linked to the Suffolk village of Bures. Two centuries before George Huntington spotted the genetic syndrome, Sydenham's interest was in a different type of chorea known as St Vitus's dance, which he realized to be in some cases a complication of rheumatic fever. He distinguished this 'common' chorea from the epidemic variety that had been seen in outbreaks during the Middle Ages, which was sometimes taken as evidence of possession but would now be attributed to mass hysteria. Of all Sydenham's proposals and innovations, only this one still celebrates his name: Sydenham's chorea is an unexplained neurological after-effect of rheumatic fever, itself a late product of streptococcal infections of the throat and the skin, just the sort of illnesses that Sydenham used to write about.

It took only a decade to produce the writings that launched a new era in medicine. Sydenham was sixty-four when his final work appeared but he ended by admitting something few great men ever

confess, that he had no more to say on his subject, that he had now
written everything he knew about medicine. With that, and with no
further comments in print, he died.

Round St James's Park and past Westminster Abbey I walked, quick-
ening my pace in the rain that had begun with the first fading of
daylight. It seemed as if it had been raining constantly since I set out
on my journey. Despite holding a newspaper over my head like an
umbrella I was wet and getting wetter. My clothes were sticking to me
and once in a while I waded into a puddle I had failed to spot. On the
corner of Great Peter Street and St Anne's Street I found what I was
looking for, the Salvation Army hostel.

George Orwell, after seeing what he called the fringes of poverty
while writing *Down and Out in Paris and London*, remarked,

> I shall never again think that all tramps are drunken scoundrels, nor expect
> a beggar to be grateful when I give him a penny, nor be surprised if men out
> of work lack energy, nor subscribe to the Salvation Army . . .

The hostel in Westminster was already twenty years old when
Orwell was dossing around London, having opened in 1911 with 575
beds. Although it had been steadily reduced to 261 by the time I called,
it was still the largest Salvation Army hostel in Britain. Until ten years
ago it had one bath for all its residents. Now there was a plan to
demolish the whole building.

The man at the hostel reception showed me where to wait until the
Major arrived for our appointment; I took a seat beside a corridor. A
few of the men who lived here, and they were all men, passed without
paying me much attention. That night there were over 200 staying, an
average number: all without homes, most without jobs, many without
roots, victims in a crisis across the country, caught in a spiral of
homelessness, unemployment and ill health.

After a while I was taken on a tour of the place by the man in
day-to-day charge at Westminster, Jack Middleton, whose rank was
captain. All these ranks exactly mimicking the echelons of regular army
officers sounded odd, even vaguely sinister, in the incongruous setting
of a shelter for the homeless. But when they were first used they must

have appeared almost illustrious. It was when William Booth, giving a revivalist talk in Whitby, was billed as the 'General of the Hallelujah Army' that the military metaphor was born. In the second half of the nineteenth century to be a soldier was to be a member of a noble profession and it would have been hard to think of a more fitting comparison for those who were doing the Lord's work than those who were fighting the Queen's fight. A century later the ranks of brigadier and territorial commander seem distinctly unchristian but they are really no worse than old-fashioned. Similarly, that familiar image of the Salvationists, the brass band, was not something they planned from the start. It began when the bodyguards they initially needed to stop the public from beating them up brought along their instruments to accompany the singing. Presumably the brass oompah sounded right for a spiritual reveille, so it stayed.

The rows of residents in the first hostel lounge we came to looked like a cross-section of life on the streets. Some, with their luxuriant beards and matted hair, were caricatures of what used to be called men of the road; it seemed to me that most of them were severely mentally ill. Others had the crimson blotchy faces of heavy drinkers. A few looked different: their clothes were ordinary but one layer too light for the cold weather, they carried their trays with a steady hand and had the subdued demeanour of men who have been kicked in the teeth by circumstance.

A quarter of the folk who slept here did so all the year round and about the same number were temporary guests who might stay for weeks or months before moving on. The rest were passing through, Westminster hostel being the first stop for migrants from outside the capital. They came from anywhere in the country, including Scotland or Ireland: out of work, out of money, out of luck. Middle-aged men splitting up from their families take refuge in anonymous places; some end up licking their wounds in a Salvationists' television lounge. Those I saw had an awkward manner and a submissive look that goes with misfortune; although outside the hostel there was nothing that would mark them out as homeless, it would not have been hard to identify them as solitary.

There were two lounges, one each for BBC and ITV, but the larger one was nearly full while the other was nearly deserted, ITV being more popular because it was broadcast in the smoking room. These were also the places where religious services took place. Off the main sitting areas was the kitchen with huge fridges that could have held a small meeting, piled with boxes of food donated by some of the bigger shops around London. Most of what its residents ate, though, Captain Middleton told me, had to be bought by the hostel. It was policy to charge for half-board and the men paid for it using their housing benefit and some of their income support. Insisting on half-board guaranteed a regular income for the hostel but that was not in itself the intention; this was no holiday hotel out to make a living. By knowing how many meals would be needed the staff could buy in bulk, spend less and charge less. The system also made sure that everyone staying there was certain of two reasonable meals, by institution standards, and that no one went hungry after wasting their benefits on something less nutritious, such as drink.

Alcohol itself is banned from the premises though peaceful drunks are tolerated. 'It's the ones who stand in the corridor singing "Nellie Dean" that are asked to go,' Major Lloyd told me later. Drugs are not an overt problem; any young person with a drug habit is directed to a more suitable hostel. Was that why I had seen no one who looked much under thirty? It was true that few young men came to the Westminster hostel but drugs were not the reason. 'They're not made welcome by the older residents,' was the Major's opinion. 'The older men see the young ones as a reproach because they haven't yet given up.'

From the dormitories upstairs I could see outside to other parts of London. There was a clear view of Westminster Abbey. The building across the road was the Department of Environment, which numbered housing and homelessness among its responsibilities. Inside there were rows of beds with iron frames and lockers packed close to them. The walls were cream and the air smelled of urine and disinfectant. The long rooms were empty and the man we surprised who was washing in an adjoining bathroom turned out to be a member of staff. No one was allowed up here until mid-evening because of the risk of theft.

Orwell loathed the Salvation Army because of its rules. A whistle was blown to send people to bed, another to rouse them early next morning. Drinking was banned, of course, but so were cooking, swearing and playing cards. In some hostels he visited attendance at religious services was compulsory. 'They cannot even run a lodging house without making it stink of charity,' he wrote.

Without doubt the Salvationists began with good intentions and it seemed that by the time Orwell was one of their flock some of their initial ideas had been distorted. The army trappings that had started as a cry of evangelism had given rise, in Orwell's view, to 'semi-military discipline'. In the same way William Booth's concern for the urban poor had been corrupted. Booth considered the Church to have lost touch with its main purpose, improving the welfare of the disadvantaged. As a young man he led an occupation of the front pews in his church, reserved for the well-off, by impoverished members of the parish. In the East End of London, where he later worked, he saw alcohol as a demon because it worsened the miserable lot of the poor, turning them sick. They had no jobs, they were ill, their houses were filthy and they spent their time and what money they had in alehouses. Whole families drank heavily together and as the women became incapable of looking after their drunken children, the men became unemployable. Alcohol lubricated the cycle of illness and poverty and so sobriety was part of salvation. But gradually the hatred of drinking acquired a life of its own and needed no social justification; in Orwell's day alcohol was a self-evident evil to the Salvation Army.

The Westminster hostel itself is another relic of an earlier era when large institutions were places where you could find protection. Now they are despised as dehumanizing but in the nineteenth century they were a genuine asylum for society's rejects, most of all the insane and mentally subnormal, who are now being encouraged to go back where they came from. But it was not the institutions that were bad, not at first, because the community their inmates escaped from was by comparison a terrible place. Their current image as restrictive and impersonal misses the point of their original existence, just as the strangeness to the modern ear of the military ranks in the Salvation Army and the impression of overzealousness in its ban on drink are only half the picture, omitting the reason that such oddities were once thought to be worthwhile.

The Salvationists have belatedly caught up with the times. The rules are few and the moral disapproval of alcohol is more a ban on rowdiness. Smaller hostels and special houses for certain groups of people – the elderly and the young, for instance – have taken over from the massive shelters like Westminster and its duplicate that used to stand across the Thames at Blackfriars, which was demolished a couple of years ago. The building I was in would soon be following suit and no one could have been happier to see it go than the Captain who ran it.

I was led through the cavernous dormitories and down more stairs; there seemed to be no end to the angles and off-shoots of the sleeping quarters; back at ground level we reached a room where new arrivals were de-loused in a deep bath with a faecal smell and another where medical checks were carried out. By this time the Major had joined us. He was a smart, sturdy man with an air that was certainly semi-military and a crisp uniform that would not have been out of place in nearby New Scotland Yard. He talked about his work with the kind of bluntness that can seem harsh but is really a reflection of the hard-edged compassion that people need in order to be effective in his line of business. He told me about the hostel's medical services.

Illness is part of life on the streets. Chest infections are common and tuberculosis is a risk made more likely by alcohol. Conditions that need continual monitoring, such as diabetes or epilepsy, can easily go untreated. The mentally ill accumulate in places like this. Major Lloyd made no pretence of offering health care: 'Nurses visit our diabetics. Psychiatric nurses will give schizophrenics their drugs. Our care assistants can make sure that people take their pills. We keep an eye on anyone who is sick. But we don't do any therapeutic work. Our facilities are for housing re-settlement.'

'Do you find much mental illness here?'

'We see two groups of people. There are the ones the hospitals discharge. And there are the men who come here because they have left their families, the ones who haven't been homeless before. The divorcees go mad here. They can't take it.'

In the East End there is a house for drying out alcoholics. A mobile

X-ray unit tours the London hostels detecting tuberculosis. 'We tell the men to have the X-ray or go somewhere else,' said Major Lloyd. But help from hospitals and doctors has been hard to win.

'They didn't want much to do with us twenty years ago,' recalled the Major. 'If one of the men was ill, we would ring for an ambulance and they would tell us they wouldn't come unless the man had seen a GP. So we would phone round all the local GPs but none of them would come here. In the end we used to leave whoever was ill on the pavement outside and dial 999 to say that someone had just collapsed in the street beside the hostel. That was the only way to get help.'

Now the Westminster hostel has its own doctor, a volunteer who calls every week. 'He's been coming for years, ever since he read about our problems getting medical back-up. He had bought some fish and chips and while he was eating them he saw an article about the Salvation Army in the paper they were wrapped in. The article complained about the lack of support from doctors so he rang us that night.'

It was the kind of story the Salvationists love: a conversion experience. Major Lloyd had his own tale on the same theme and he told it with a well-practised fluency though it was no less impressive for that.

'My mother died when I was eight, in 1949. We lived in Middlesbrough and my father worked in a steel foundry. It was shift work, and he was away from six till two or two till ten or for the night shift. And he was a boozer, replenishing the sweat he lost from working beside the furnaces. I never saw him. By the time I was sixteen I was drinking and I had had numerous jobs. I came to London and slept out. It was a cold night in October. A policeman said I should go to the Salvation Army at Westminster. I knew nothing about them at that time, except that they sold the *War Cry* in pubs.'

In those days the hostel still had several hundred beds and its entrance was not the easily ignored side door I had found. 'It had forbidding gates and looked worse than a prison. The yard outside was packed and there were queues everywhere to get in for a bed. I was standing in line when a Salvation Army officer came over and asked "What can I do to help you?" I was interviewed the next day and given a job as a tea boy, serving 1,500 mugs in two hours. I saw the life of the major in charge, with his family living here, and at one of the services I declared my membership in front of four hundred men.'

Over the next two decades he followed his calling. He trained as a minister of religion, rose through the ranks of the Salvationists and returned to the Westminster hostel as the Major. 'As I was getting out of my car on my first day, one of the residents said to me, "I remember you when you were nothing." I said, "I'm still nothing – what have you done?" '

The pay the Salvationists receive is not much and they retire on small pensions but I believed the Major when he said that if only one person had benefited from his work in the last thirty years, it had been worth it. He laughed when I suggested there might be other rewards, like gratitude. 'Would you be grateful?', he said. 'Why should anyone be grateful when life has done him down and he's ended up in a dump like this?'

It was easy to see that the Salvation Army had its feet on the ground, that despite the brass buttons and the anachronistic military metaphor it knew what life was like for the homeless and it went about offering them food and shelter without being either judgemental or naïve. Like most organizations engaged in decent charitable work, it was just doing the best it could, expecting a lot of itself but not much of anyone else. And its soldiers, if they were like Major Lloyd, were humane and shrewd in the same breath. But I couldn't leave without asking him about George Orwell. He hadn't read him but he showed no surprise when I told him what Orwell had disliked.

'What do you think about all the rules? And the whistle they used to blow to send people to bed?'

'In a place like this you have to have order and discipline.'

'And the compulsory religion?'

'Often the hostels had only one room so the men had to go out if they didn't want to stay for the meeting. It may sound wrong now but for some it was a life-changing experience. I didn't want to go to the meetings when I first stayed here. But it was there that I took the Christian religion and that changed my life. Otherwise I might still have been a bum on the streets. How many men don't change their lives because we are now liberal?'

The subject was ripe for argument, but it had come to a natural, rhetorical pause and, preferring to leave, I stepped into the London evening. It was dark now and cold and the streets were soaked although the rain had stopped. Down-river and past Whitehall, in the doorways of the Strand, the teenagers and psychotic homeless who were bedding down for the night were wrapping up in cardboard: to them the fresh evening threatened a freezing night. I doubled back and turned down the side of Charing Cross Station and through the Embankment underground to Hungerford Bridge, which takes pedestrians and trains from one side of the Thames to the other. It was near here that Isambard Kingdom Brunel was helping out on his father's construction of a tunnel under the river when he was injured by falling rock. As I had seen in Bristol, the result of his convalescent musings was the Clifton Suspension Bridge.

This was the end of my journey, looking into the filthy Thames at night, all thought drowned out by the trains passing a few metres away. I had set out to see the country and to explore medicine past and present, and if there were going to be any conclusions, this was the time to draw them. But were there any?

I had seen how water had bound together this clutch of islands and their health. It was the sea that had brought plague to Dorset and cholera to London via the ports in the north. It was the sea that had led to the illnesses and itches of Lowestoft fishermen. And without the healing power of water Scarborough, Bath and Walsingham would not exist. I had seen also how closely illnesses had reflected the ways people earned their living, in agriculture, in coal and lead mines, in cotton factories, in nuclear power.

It had been evident too that the fashions and achievements of medicine were inseparable from historical events. Whole dynasties had hinged on unlikely cures and probable placebos starting with King Bladud and his disease-ridden pigs. William of Orange had invaded after Bath solved the infertility of James and Mary of Modena; Thomas Sydenham had finally settled for medicine after the Restoration put paid to his politics. Equally the ties between health and the Church were close; I had witnessed the influence of religion in Belfast, on Harris and in a Salvation Army hostel. That medicine was entwined with the culture of the country could not have been clearer.

But walking across Hungerford Bridge to my car I did not feel as if the journey was over. I had been marooned in the Hebrides; I had trudged round a coal-mine; I had walked in a murderous part of West Belfast; I had even been evicted from a campsite near Scarborough; and yet there was something about this ending that made me want to continue, a feeling that something was unfinished.

I suppose it was that, just as medicine had no real boundaries, the stories I had uncovered through their medical connections were themselves part of a broader narrative. Wherever I left off, several more trails were untouched. And in this the tales I had collected had something in common with how I had found them – with travel.

Every journey misses countless possible routes because of those it chooses to take. And no matter where and when you stop, you can also start there on another trip. Which is why a bridge seems always a fitting place to end: you can arrive at one side and leave at the other as if setting out again. It is also why travel, although it can be uncomfortable, lonely and exhausting, can be so compelling a habit: because no journey is ever quite complete. Like the conversation I had recently left in a run-down Salvationist shelter, it merely comes to a natural pause.

Acknowledgements

A BOOK like this is inevitably written with a certain amount of artistic licence. Some visits were made twice to check facts; although they all seem to have been made alone, on some I was accompanied; and there was a long gap in the middle when I wrote nothing and travelled nowhere. There is no shame in this sort of distortion: a number of seamless travel books are based on piecemeal travel. Even Orwell, I am told, while writing *Down and Out in Paris and London* took time off from London's streets to allow himself a few home comforts.

The historical passages too are, to the best of my knowledge, accurate but not necessarily the whole story. I have used mainly secondary sources rather than original manuscripts: this is not meant as a work of scholarship. The books I have borrowed from are listed below.

Lists of thanks can be tedious but not to acknowledge certain people would be negligent. The first of these is my partner Juliet Haselden, who helped develop my poorly formed ideas, read what I had written and came with me on half the journey. The next is Dr Adrian Caro who unselfishly lent me his Ph.D. thesis, a rich source of genealogical data on Huntington's chorea. My sister Carolyn and her partner David provided me with literary advice and allowed me to borrow their car to go to Harris, an act I rewarded by backing it into a ditch. Julian Loose and Roger Osborne of Faber and Faber were an important source of encouragement and comment.

The following people helped me in one way or another and none expected any repayment: Dr Chris Abell, Dr Stefan Cembrowicz, Dr Sudhamony Chatterjee, Dr Sarah Crook, Dr Peter Curran, Brian Davies, Catherine Floyd, Lyn Gardner, Mick Grant, Hutch and colleagues, Major Keith Lloyd, Dr Gerry Loughrey, Dr Graeme McDonald, Dr Philip McGarry, Dr Liz McWhirter, Captain Jack Middleton, Bob Neil, Jo Oldman and his father, Dr John Robertson, Dr Roy Robertson, Lynda Thomas, Shirley Williams, Len Willies, Dr Robin Wood.

My sources of historical information were numerous, some providing a single fact, others an entire life story. An invaluable book for general background and specific points was *A Social History of Medicine* by F. F. Cartwright (Longman, 1977); another was *Disease, Medicine and Society in England 1550–1860* by Roy Porter (Macmillan, 1987). Many of the biographical books I used were found in the library at the Wellcome Institute for the History of Medicine, London. Overall I perused everything from tourist brochures to scientific papers to find the kind of details I could use; I also expanded on ideas I had touched on in the *British Medical Journal*, vol. 297 (1988) and vol. 298 (1989), on the Outer Hebrides and the Salvation Army respectively, and in the *Bulletin of the Royal College of Psychiatrists*, vol. 14 (1990), on mad cow disease.

The quotations I have used came from the following:

IDRIS DAVIS, 'Gwalia Deserta' from *The Collected Poems of Idris Davis*, edited by Islwyn Jenkins, 2nd edn, Gomer Press, Llandysul,1980.

DANIEL DEFOE, *A Tour through the Whole Island of Great Britain*, Penguin Books, Harmondsworth, 1986.

CHARLES DICKENS, *Hard Times*, Penguin Books, Harmondsworth, 1985.

JOHN ENTWISLE, 'Light upon dark places', *Bolton Journal*, 1884.

MICHAEL FOOT, *Aneurin Bevan*, vol. 1, 1897–1945, Granada, London, 1982.

GEORGE HUNTINGTON, *Journal of Nervous and Mental Disease*, vol. 37, 1910, p.255.

JOHN LIVY, *Report of the Health of Bolton During the Year 1873*, Borough of Bolton, 1873.

LOUIS MACNEICE, 'Carrickfergus' in *Louis MacNeice: Selected Poems*, edited by Michael Longley, Faber & Faber, London, 1988.

GEORGE ORWELL, *Down and Out in Paris and London*, Penguin Books, Harmondsworth, 1977.

J. B. PRIESTLEY, *English Journey*, Penguin Books, Harmondsworth, 1987.

HALLIDAY SUTHERLAND, *Hebridean Journey*, Geoffrey Bles, London, 1939.

WILLIAM WEBB, *British Medical Journal*, 15 August 1857.

In addition to these, my other sources of information were:

G. W. BARNES and THOMAS STEVENS, *The History of the Clifton Suspension Bridge*, 19th edn, The Clifton Suspension Bridge Trust, Bristol, 1977.

GEORGINA BATTISCOMBE, *Shaftesbury: a Biography of the 7th Earl, 1801–1885*, Constable, London, 1974.

D. BLACK *Investigation of the Possible Increased Incidence of Cancer in West Cumbria: Report of the Independent Advisory Group*, Her Majesty's Stationery Office, London, 1984.

ALAN BOLD, *Bonnie Prince Charlie*, Pitkin Pictorials, London, 1973.

ARTHUR BOND, *The Walsingham Story through 900 Years*, 2nd edn, The Guild Shop, Walsingham, 1988.

E. M. BROCKBANK, *Mulespinner's Cancer*, H. K. Lewis & Co., London, 1941.

G. W. BROWN and R. PRUDO. 'Psychiatric disorder in a rural and an urban population: 1. Aetiology of depression.' *Psychological Medicine*, vol. 11, 1981, p.581.

JOHN G. CLIFFORD, *Eyam Plague 1665–1666*, John G. Clifford, Eyam, 1989.

DAVID COHEN and LIZ MCWHIRTER, 'War and peace', in *The Power of Psychology*, edited by D. Cohen, Croom Helm, London, 1987.

RICHARD COLLIER, *The General next to God*, Fontana/Collins, London, 1968.

G. J. DRAPER, C. A. STILLER, R. A. CARTWRIGHT, A. W. CRAFT and T. J. VINCENT, 'Cancer in Cumbria and in the vicinity of the Sellafield nuclear installation, 1963–90', *British Medical Journal*, vol. 306, 1993, p.89.

D. L. EMBLEM, *Peter Mark Roget: The Word and the Man*, Longman, Harlow, 1970.

JOHN ENTWISLE, *A Report Of The Sanatory Condition Of The Borough Of Bolton*, Bolton, 1848.

M. J. GARDNER, A. J. HALL, S. DOWNES and J. D. TERRELL, 'Follow up study of children born elsewhere but attending schools in Seascale, West Cumbria (schools cohort)', *British Medical Journal*, vol. 295, 1987, p. 819.

M. J. GARDNER, M. P. SNEE, A. J. HALL, C. A. POWELL, S. DOWNES and J. D. TERRELL, 'Results of case-control study of leukaemia and lymphoma among young people near Sellafield Nuclear Plant in West Cumbria', *British Medical Journal*, vol. 300, 1990, p.423.

PAUL HARKER, *Communicable Disease Report 1991*, West Dorset Health Authority, Dorchester, 1992.

GLYNN HARRISON, DAVID OWENS, ANTHONY HOLDEN, DAVID NIELSEN and DAPHNE BOOT, 'A prospective study of severe mental disorder in Afro-Caribbean patients', *Psychological Medicine*, vol. 18, 1988, p. 643.

W. H. HATTIE, 'Huntington's chorea', *American Journal of Insanity*, vol. 66, 1909, p. 123.

ELY LIEBOW, *Dr Joe Bell, Model For Sherlock Holmes*, Bowling Green University Popular Press, Bowling Green, Ohio, 1982.

M. M. LINEHAN, J. L. GOODSTEIN and S. L. NIELSEN, 'Reasons for staying alive when you are thinking of killing yourself: the reason for living inventory', *Journal of Counselling and Clinical Psychology*, vol. 51, 1983, p. 276.

HENRY LONSDALE, *Life of Robert Knox, the Anatomist*, MacMillan, London, 1870.

J. R. MCLAUGHLIN, T. W. ANDERSON, E. A. CLARKE and W. KING, *Occupational Exposure of Fathers to Ionising Radiation and the Risk of Leukaemia in Offspring: a Case-control Study*, Atomic Energy Control Board (Ottawa), 1992.

LIZ MCWHIRTER and KAREN TREW, 'Children in Northern Ireland: a lost generation?' in *The Child in His Family*, vol. 7, edited by E. James Anthony and Colette Chiland, John Wiley & Sons, London, 1982.

O. ODEGAARD, 'Emigration and insanity', *Acta Psychiatrica Scandinavica*, Supplement 4, 1932.

GEORGE ORWELL, *The Road To Wigan Pier*, Penguin Books, Harmondsworth, 1989.

ISOBEL RAE, *Knox: The Anatomist*, Oliver & Boyd, Edinburgh and London, 1964.

J. R. ROBERTSON, A. B. V. BUCKNALL, P. D. WELSBY, J. J. K. ROBERTS, J. M. INGLIS, J. F. PEUTHERER and R. P. BRETTLE, 'Epidemic of AIDS related virus (HTLV-III/LAV) infection among intravenous drug users', *British Medical Journal*, vol. 292, 1986, p.527.

J. R. ROBERTSON, C. A. SKIDMORE and J. K. K. ROBERTS, 'The dynamics of an illicit drug scene', *Scottish Medical Journal*, vol. 33, 1988, p.293.

H. HAROLD SCOTT, *Some Notable Epidemics*, Edward Arnold, London, 1934.

MYRTLE SIMPSON, *Simpson the Obstetrician*, Gollancz, London, 1972.

C. A. SKIDMORE, J. R. ROBERTSON, A. A. ROBERTSON and R. A.

ELTON, 'After the epidemic: follow up study of HIV seroprevalence and changing patterns of drug use', *British Medical Journal*, vol. 300, 1990, p.219.

PAUL WALKER, *Norwich and District: On the State of its Health 1988*, vol. 1, Norwich and District Health Authority, Norwich, 1989.

E. MARJORIE WALLACE, *The First Vaccinator: Benjamin Jesty of Yetminster and Worth Matravers and his Family*, E. Marjorie Wallace, Worth Matravers, 1981.

JOHN K. WALTON, *The English Seaside Resort: a Social History 1750–1914*, Leicester University Press, Leicester, 1983.

CECIL WOODHAM-SMITH, *Florence Nightingale*, Constable, London, 1950.

PHILIP ZIEGLER, *The Black Death*, Penguin Books, Harmondsworth, 1982.

Index